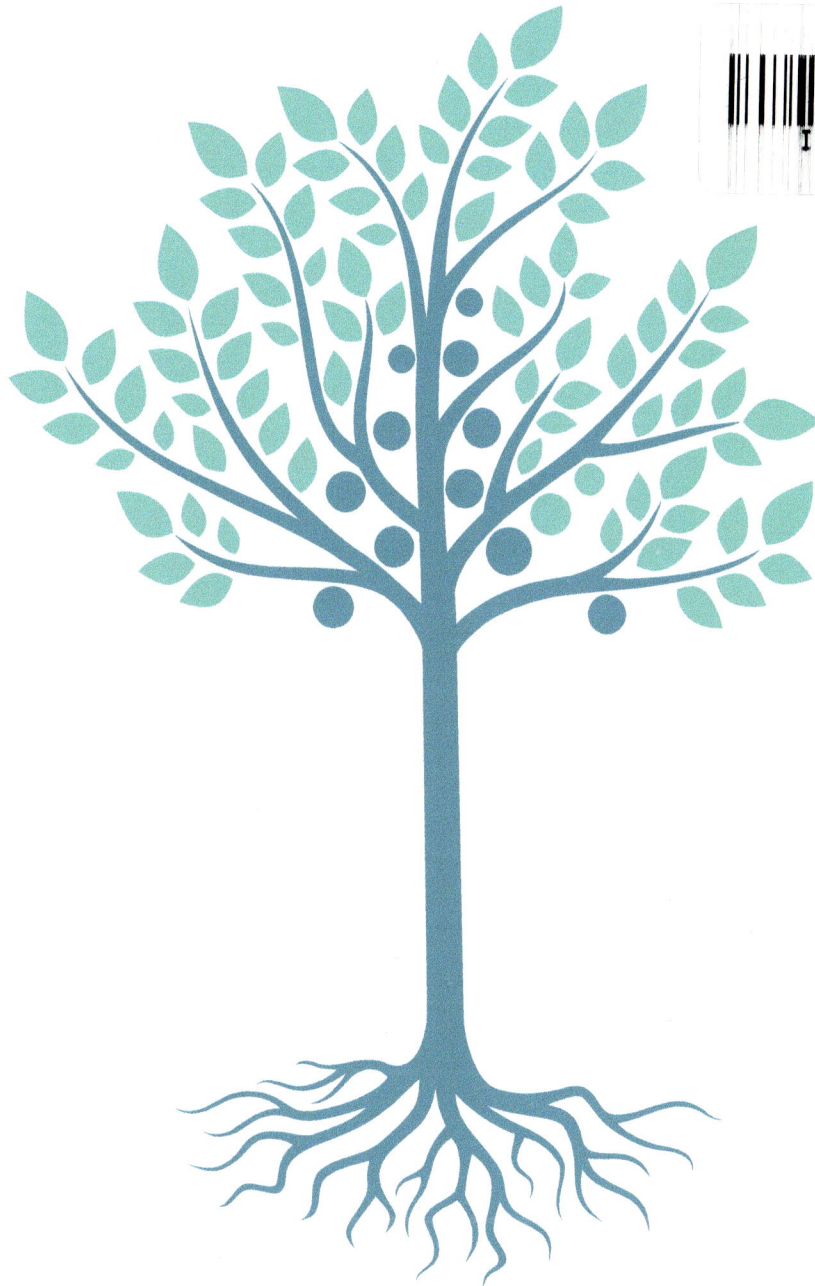

Hope for Healing WORKBOOK
Creating Therapeutic Partnerships

Kara Ware, NBC-HWC
with Paula Kruppstadt, MD

"Healing isn't something you do, it's who you become." Kara Ware

To learn more about Kara Ware, visit karawarecoaching.com.

Contributions by Functional Pediatrician, Paula Kruppstadt, MD

To learn more about Dr. Paula Kruppstadt (Dr. K) and Hope for Healing, visit https://get2theroot.com/pediatric-providers/

Cover photos:
Man with children: o_shumilova/Shutterstock.com
Woman with boy: Altanaka/Shutterstock.com
Family at dinner table: Monkey Business Images/Shutterstock.com

Waterfall photo copyright kavram via Creative Market

First printing, 2023

ISBN: 978-1-955791-41-0

Ordering information: Special discounts are available on quantity purchases by bookstores, corporations, associations, and others. For details, contact the publisher at:

sales@braughlerbooks.com
or at 937-58-BOOKS

For questions or comments about this book, please write to:

info@braughlerbooks.com

Braughler™
Books
braughlerbooks.com

Contents

Foreword

Heartbreak, Grief, Loss, Transforming, Joy

In 2004, when my son regressed into Autism, I experienced debilitating heartbreak and grief. I grieved for the loss of my child. I wept for his obvious pain. I mourned for my youngest son. I grieved for the loss of my own freedom, health, sleep, marriage, and the loss of my life's dream. Because I had no choice, I kept waking up in the morning.

After our first biomed doctor's appointment, in March 2006, where I learned of his toxicity, leaky gut, mineral and vitamin deficiencies, hormonal and immune dysregulation, and viral, bacterial, fungal, and parasite load, I was in a full-blown state of emotional crisis. As I drove home from that three-hour appointment, shock set in. I was jolted back to reality by the blaring horn and bright lights of driving into oncoming traffic. The next thing I remember, I was in a ditch on the opposite side of the road. I began violently heaving when an uncontrolled wail came forth, followed by my body convulsing with sobs. I remember realizing I was hyperventilating because we were safe; I would have rather us all die at that moment. Life was THAT HORRIBLE.

I was overcome by grief, guilt, and shame for having had these thoughts. How could I ever contemplate such atrocities? But I now understand how common those feelings are. If you have thoughts like this, it doesn't make you a bad person or parent. It makes you human.

Chronic conditions and devastating developmental delays want to consume all of you; mentally, emotionally, physically, and spiritually. They want to take over everything and drive you to feel defeated and, at its darkest, contemplate the unthinkable. You must learn to become more than your circumstances to affect positive change. **Healing is not something you do; it's who you become**. To heal the physical body, you must go further upstream and deprogram old beliefs and thoughts that, up until now, have been guiding your feelings, emotions, decisions, words, actions, and habits. I encourage you to place priority on the mental, emotional, and spiritual facets of healing to build new beliefs and thoughts that create elevated emotions that regulate hormones and modulate gene expression to drive different decisions, words, actions, and habits to produce different results. You have the most power to influence your healing journey by training your mind and emotions. When you assume responsibility for your mindset, emotional intelligence, and habits, partner with a functional medicine provider, and stick with the process, profound healing occurs!

So, as you begin to work with this curriculum, I advise this... make your change process all about what you value, love, and treasure the most rather than about battling the dis-ease. Make your change process about becoming a more courageous, resilient, radiant version of yourself. Allow it to be a journey of building happiness and joy in the throes of great adversity. Your mind and emotions are powerful; train them to work for you rather than against you and **YOU WILL DO** what many still say is impossible.

Paula Kruppstadt, MD, Chief Medical Officer of Hope for Healing, a pediatric and primary care functional medicine practice, has collaborated with me throughout the pages of this workbook. I highly recommend you choose to partner with her team to move toward restoring balance and function to your own life.

In solidarity and friendship,

Kara

All roads lead to Hope

Dear Patients,

We are grateful you have decided to partner with our team at Hope for Healing.

Our vision is to see every member of the Hope for Healing community—patients and staff—**thrive.**

Regardless of age or experience, we believe that a vibrant, high-quality life consists of *physical, mental, emotional, and spiritual health*.

In order to see our vision become a reality in the lives of each of our patients, our mission is to equip you with the education, like-minded community, and therapeutic partnership needed to optimize your whole-being health beyond the absence of disease, transform hopelessness into hope and experience profound healing and restoration.

We all do better in community. In order to heal and maintain an optimal quality of life, it is our belief that patients need a network of support and a *like-minded* community to connect and collaborate with. Additionally, Hope for Healing's mission is to make functional medicine more affordable and accessible to best serve the numerous patients who are looking to our team to help reverse complex disease states and prevent symptoms of imbalance. Therefore, group visits and community outreach events are a part of our patient experience.

"Of all the diseases I have known, loneliness is the worst." Mother Teresa

---

After nearly two decades of practice experience, we have learned the most efficient and effective way to walk with you through your unique journey is by taking you through the functional medicine approach in an intelligent sequence: Lifestyle | Genetics | Medical.

Lifestyle modifications are the bedrock of functional medicine and are required to enhance your return on investment on out-of-pocket medical visits, diagnostic labs, supplements, and functional interventions. Therefore, health coaches are a part of your care team.

By evaluating the role that interactions among genetic, environmental, and lifestyle factors have played in contributing to your or your child's current state of imbalance (chronic illness, etc.), you will gain the knowledge needed to strategically alter your lifestyle and reverse the effects of these factors.

"Guided learning is much more efficient than trial and error."
Dr. James Prochaska

This workbook aims to design your comprehensive and coordinated family care plan and implement and sustain lifestyle modifications (nutrition, sleep, stress, relationships, movement, finances, and time management) that match your current ability. Placing priority on establishing, revisiting, and strengthening this foundation before layering in advanced medical protocols activates you in the healing partnership with your medical providers. Functional medicine is a mutual-participatory medical model where patients and providers work together as **equal therapeutic partners**.

The next step in your patient journey is to meet with our genetic provider. Without genetics, we are all flying blind. Genetic testing provides you with evidence-based, personalized action steps based on your unique biological makeup to ensure that any recommendations made are both necessary and effective. Genetics is the missing puzzle piece in the medical mystery cases of many patients, the guide to preventative care, and a key tool for those seeking to optimize their health and performance.

Focusing on the lifestyle and genetics before meeting with your medical provider is how we use your time and financial investment wisely and expedite your healing. With these crucial steps to your healing journey already completed, you and your medical provider will be able to get started healing the underlying imbalances that are creating your symptoms.

A note to our families living with Autism, PANS/PANDAS

Whether you are here as the patient or are here because your child is the patient, we all must actively learn how to write, implement, sustain, and tell our stories. If you are a parent, you cannot ask your child to participate in any lifestyle changes that you are unwilling to do for yourself. You must lead by example. Recovering a child from Autism and PANS/PANDAS is a journey we take with them, not something we do to them. Please take this opportunity to be a part of your child's care by going through your own healing journey!

A note to our teenage patients

Your parents and our team at Hope for Healing are here to help. However, we need your participation. We ask that you join the group coaching classes with your parents and focus on what you can do. You will also be present at the one-to-one coaching session to further learn what is causing your symptoms. You will walk away from this coaching session with a plan that empowers you to implement the changes that you feel confident and competent to achieve.

Every one of the medical providers at Hope for Healing has been extensively trained and mentored in the principles and practices of functional medicine. I trust each one of our providers and I ask that you do the same. As the chief medical officer at Hope for Healing, I oversee the team of medical providers delivering your care. Our providers work together to deliver the highest level and quality of care to each of our patients. Behind the scenes, our medical team meets on a regular basis to collaborate and consult with one another regarding each patient's case, continuing medical education, and discussing the latest research, treatment, and health-optimization findings. In order to deliver personalized, evidence-based care to our patients, we are committed to consistent growth and learning. Hope for Healing recognizes the gap between the latest research and the integration of this research into medical practice.

Functional Medicine is a Process *aka* a Journey. It's advisable to prepare and pack for this journey with patience, curiosity, and a mind open to strategize outside of your comfort zone. Our team assists you in the strategy; however, we emphasize the importance for you to be patient with yourself, your healing process, and our team. Your symptoms took time to show up; likewise, it will take time for your symptoms to be placed into remission as we address the root cause(s) of your health challenges. Please read the Memorandum of Understanding that is included with your new patient paperwork and sign an agreement to treat our **entire** team with patience, respect, and kindness as we partner with you on your healing journey.

I believe that there's always a way to recover. There's always a way to get better. Please place top priority on these lifestyle changes and I promise you, the road to Hope and Healing will open up with endless possibilities.

"The goal of a physician should be to find health because anyone can find disease."
Andrew Taylor Still, DO

With much gratitude,

"Dr. K"

PS When you or your child begins to feel better, please continue with your recommended medical visits. It's a long journey to repair, rebalance, and restore proper functionality if you have been sick for a long time.

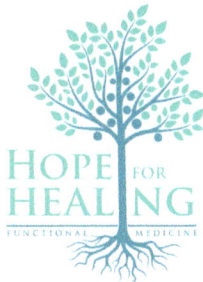

Achieve your health goals by optimizing all aspects of wellness, immunity, and longevity. Find and fix the root causes of these problems permanently.

281-725-6767 • get2theroot.com

1801 Binz Street, Suite 400 • Houston, Texas • 77004

121 Vision Park Blvd #200 • Shenandoah, Texas • 77384

hope@get2theroot.com

Glossary of Terms

Functional medicine has a vocabulary that is important for patients to learn so you are speaking the same language with your care team. You will find below the vocabulary words elaborated on in the Medical Interventions section of your workbook. We have tried to put these definitions into layman's terms.

Actinomycetes (Actinos): a type of bacteria found on/in the human body, in water-damaged buildings, and throughout nature (soil species). Some are pathogenic and cause disease, and some do not. Actinos are like a cross between a bacterium and a fungus. They form a biofilm, like a bomb shelter, around themselves to protect themselves and make it hard for the immune system to find and destroy them.

Adaptive Immune System: the side of our immune system that makes antibodies and is **not** present at birth. Antibodies help us fight off foreign invaders. These foreign invaders are called antigens. When we are given a traditional vaccine, our adaptive immune system makes antibodies. Additionally, when we have an infection, such as chickenpox, we make antibodies to that virus (antigens presented). If those antibodies are robust (you can test by drawing blood), then you won't need to "boost" the adaptive immune system by getting the chickenpox vaccine.

Antecedent: factors, genetic or acquired, that predispose to illness.

Autonomic Nervous System: the part of the nervous system responsible for the control of the bodily functions not consciously directed, such as breathing, the heartbeat, and digestive processes. The autonomic nervous system consists of two parts: the sympathetic and parasympathetic nervous systems.

Biomarkers: specific labs, and cultures that can be measured and tracked. Many biomarkers will change with effective treatment and therapy.

Biotoxin: a toxin made by living organisms like bacteria, mold, viruses, spiders, snakes, algae, etcetera …

Blood-Brain Barrier: a "leaky gut" allows toxins into the bloodstream. Because of this, certain substances in the body that were blocked before can now cross over into the brain creating cognitive and mood symptoms. Many doctors call this phenomenon a "leaky brain." We can measure circulating antibodies directed against the brain and nervous system, proving the existence of a "leaky brain."

Brain-Heart Coherence: a state in which the heart, mind, and emotions are synchronized and balanced. This state is associated with feelings of well-being, relaxation, delight, satisfaction, and improved cognitive function.

Bristol Stool Chart: a chart used to characterize what your bowel movements look like.

CIRS: Chronic Inflammatory Response Syndrome (CIRS) is a condition that about a quarter of the population has the potential to develop worldwide. It occurs when a person is exposed to something that stimulates their INNATE immune system, especially from within a WDB (Water Damaged Building). The innate immune system responds by increasing cytokines, small messengers of inflammation. With CIRS, you cannot naturally cool your innate immune system down after exposure. 21 to 24 percent of the population has CIRS. If you look at the rates of autoimmunity, they're very similar. Triggers of CIRS are biotoxins (toxins made by living organisms like bacteria, mold, viruses, spiders, snakes, algae, etcetera).

Clostridia: bacteria that make a short-chain fatty acid called propionic acid. An abundance of propionic acid can make a person angry and emotionally labile. Clostridial overgrowth in the gut is very common in autistic children.

Current Ability: design your care plan based on your current ability (motivation + competence + confidence)

Cytokine Storm: cytokines are like policemen. They tell the white cells in our body what to do. When we get sick, typically we get a fever, we feel bad, we're tired, then our temperature goes down and we feel better. The things in our body, immune molecules that make us feel bad, are called cytokines. When a patient is dealing with recurring, unresolved infections or exposure to biotoxins, a cytokine storm takes place. A cytokine storm means runaway inflammation. If those cytokines, little invisible messengers, stay in our bodies without returning to normal levels, then our white cells (which fight the infections) lose their regulation: the white cells don't know what to do. So, you could be really sick, feel bad all the time, but "never get sick." Your "normal" way to feel is not truly healthy; many people coming to H4H "never get sick," but they feel terrible most of the time.

Dairy/ Casein/ Lactose: cows, sheep, and goats are where we traditionally get "dairy" products from. All of these dairy products have two proteins in them called casein and whey. Casein is very inflammatory to human beings unless it is in human dairy (breast milk). Lactose is a carbohydrate that is contained within dairy products. Being "lactose intolerant" is not the same thing as being allergic to milk. It means that you lack the enzymes in your intestinal tract to break down lactose. This leads to gas, abdominal pain, and in many cases diarrhea.

Dental Amalgam: the material used to make fillings for cavities caused by tooth decay. This is a mixture of metals, consisting of liquid (elemental) mercury and a powdered alloy composed of silver, tin, and copper.

Disease: Disease is a term used by the medical field to describe a collection of symptoms that generate a diagnosis. We choose to use the word dis-ease since it is indicative of your body feeling a lack of ease or comfort. Dis-ease is the state of being in need of removing, replacing, reinoculating, repairing, and rebalancing in order to help you heal what is causing the symptoms of the disease so you can experience well-being.

Dysbiosis: a condition when too many of the wrong gut bugs (parasites, yeast, protozoa, and "bad" bacteria) or not enough of the good ones (like Lactobacillus or Bifidobacterium) are in your gut, which can lead to serious damage to your health.

Emotional Intelligence: Emotional intelligence (otherwise known as emotional quotient or EQ) is the ability to understand, use, and manage your own emotions in positive ways to relieve stress, communicate effectively, empathize with others, overcome challenges, and diffuse conflict.

Enteric Nervous System (ENS): is a network of sensory neurons, motor neurons, and interneurons embedded in the wall of the gastrointestinal system, extending from the lower third of the esophagus to the rectum and classified as a branch of the autonomic nervous system, alongside the sympathetic and parasympathetic branches. The ENS is called the "second brain."

Epigenetics: the study of how your behaviors and environment can cause changes that affect how your genes work. Epigenetic changes are modifications to DNA that regulate whether genes are turned on or off. Unlike genetic mutations that create predictable disease states, epigenetic changes are reversible and do not change your DNA sequence but can change how your body expresses what a DNA sequence is saying.

ERMI: Environmental Relative Moldiness Index is a test that analyses a sample of dust from a home. The sample is analyzed using a very specific DNA-based method for quantifying mold species and the score is called the ERMI. This looks at thirty-six mold species.

Glutathione: (pronounced gloota-thigh-own) is the body's most important molecule to prevent disease and stay healthy. It's the master anti-inflammatory and master antioxidant.

Gut-Brain Axis: Many scientists have begun to refer to the gut as our second brain, an idea that is reflected in amazing books like *The Good Gut*, *Brainmaker*, *The Microbiome Solution*, *The Gut Balance Revolution*, and *The Second Brain*.

Helicobacter Pylori: little bacteria shaped like a corkscrew that has the potential to cause ulcers and gastric (stomach) and esophageal cancer. It's called a spirochete and burrows into your stomach wall and esophagus.

HERTSMI-2: This is an acronym for Health Effects Roster of Type-Specific Formers of Mycotoxins and Inflammagens, second version. This differs from the ERMI in that it looks only at five specific mold species.

Herxheimer Reaction: Drs. Jarisch and Herxheimer originally described this reaction, "Herxing", which occurs when injured or dead bacteria release their endotoxins into the blood and tissues faster than the body can comfortably handle it. This provokes a sudden and exaggerated inflammatory response. The Herxheimer Reaction is a short-term (from days to a few weeks) detoxification reaction in the body. As the body detoxifies, it is not uncommon to experience flu-like symptoms including headache, joint and muscle pain, body aches, sore throat, general malaise, sweating, chills, nausea, or other symptoms. (The death of parasites, viruses, mold, and fungi can also cause a Herxheimer reaction).

HLA Haplotype: 21 to 24 percent of the population has a genetic predisposition to developing biotoxin illness when they're exposed to a toxin from any kind of living organism. There are five separate genes that make patients susceptible to mold biotoxins diseases. The five genes we test for are HLA DRB1, DRB3, DRB4, DRB5, and DQB1.

Homeostasis: balance.

Imbalance: occurs when the function of one or more of the seven core physiological processes is not functioning correctly. This is where the term functional medicine comes from. When the function of one system is off, it often causes one or more of the other systems to dysfunction, resulting in illness. This is because all of the processes and systems in our body work together rather than independently.

Immune Dysregulation: when our white cells have high levels of cytokines around them all the time and then they don't know what to do. That's called dysregulation.

Inflammation: it is known that all chronic ailments (cardiovascular disease, migraine headaches, chronic pain, and autoimmune disorders such as rheumatoid arthritis, Hashimoto's thyroiditis, lupus, and psoriasis) are inflammatory in nature. Functional medicine seeks to identify and heal the causes of the inflammation. Inflammation is a natural response of the immune system to a foreign invader such as a virus. Chronic inflammation occurs when the immune system is not functioning properly and leads to chronic illness.

Innate Immune System: the immune system we are born with. If your innate (natural) immune system is on fire, then you should consider delaying vaccines until it is calmed/cooled down. The innate immune system provides an immediate response to foreign invaders as the fundamental "first responder" and does not have to be "taught" to respond through exposure to an invader.

Leaky Gut: described as an increase in the permeability of the intestinal lining/mucosa, which could allow bacteria, toxic digestive metabolites, bacterial toxins, and small molecules to "leak" into the bloodstream, igniting an immune response. This can affect mood, memory, cognition, focus, concentration, causing potential food sensitivities, and may lead to diarrhea/constipation/abdominal pain and bloating. Essentially, "bad stuff" is allowed to flow freely into your bloodstream.

Low Dose Naltrexone (LDN): a medication that is *not addictive*. It is an opioid antagonist; it is not an opioid. It temporarily binds to the opioid receptors that are all over a person's body to block the production of cytokines. The opioid receptors start to produce endorphins and metenkephalins after the LDN is released. Using LDN decreases inflammation in the body by modulating Toll-Like Receptors and is especially useful in autoimmune illnesses.

Mediator: ongoing exposures, factors, biochemical or psychosocial, that contribute to pathological changes and dysfunctional responses.

Microbiome: think of your gut as a garden full of flora and fauna. We are home to more than 500 different species of microbes. Some of them help us, but others are harmful.

Mind-Body Medicine: uses the power of thoughts and emotions to influence physical health.

Mold/Biotoxin Illness: you can have biotoxin illness from water damage in your home. The toxins made from bacteria and mold lead to cytokine production. You can also develop biotoxin illness from the venom of a snake or a spider.

MSH: Melanocyte Stimulating Hormone. This neuroregulatory peptide (think of it like a hormone) is made by the hypothalamus and it's released from the pituitary gland (both of these structures are in the brain). This is the beginning of the pathway that activates the expression of the genetic vulnerability to mold biotoxin illness. When MSH goes low, your natural endorphin production goes down, in addition to melatonin. When endorphins go low, you tend to develop physical pain and mental "brain" pain (think chronic pain, fibromyalgia). In children, they'll usually complain of prolonged growing pains that occur at least every other day for 1 month. The "growing pains" are not associated with exercise or activity that they completed. When endorphins go down, it's very easy to become depressed, anxious, panicked, and to develop insomnia. More often than not, adults and children with low MSH will be very tired, but when they try to sleep, they state that their brain is "wired, yet tired." When MSH goes down, it can also give you what's called a leaky gut (see definition above).

Multiple Antibiotic Resistant Coagulase Negative Staph (MARCoNS): these bacteria may infect and colonize the upper nasal passages of people, especially if their MSH (melanocyte-stimulating hormone) is low. This bacteria produces a biotoxin and drives down MSH, causing a "leaky brain" and a "leaky gut."

Neuroplasticity: also known as neural plasticity, or brain plasticity, is the ability of neural networks in the brain to change through growth and reorganization.

Nonviolent Communication (NVC): violent strategies, whether verbal or physical, are learned behaviors taught and supported by the prevailing culture. A technique for you to practice is gathering facts through observing without evaluating, genuinely and concretely expressing feelings and needs, and formulating effective and empathetic requests. Practicing NVC makes it much easier to talk about solutions that satisfy all parties.

Nutraceutical: a food containing health-giving additives and having medicinal benefits.

Parasympathetic Nervous System: restores the body to a state of calm and inhibits the body from overworking. It helps to restore the body to a composed state of "rest and digest."

Pharmacogenomics: Adverse drug reactions are the 5th leading cause of death in the United States today. Genetic factors account for up to 95% of an individual's drug response. For over 20 years, the field of pharmacogenomics (PGx) has been developing to provide insight into how each person's unique genetic profile affects how the medication will work for them.

Physiological Processes: are the ways in which organ systems, organs, tissues, cells, and biomolecules work together to accomplish the complex goal of sustaining life. Physiological mechanisms are the smaller physical and chemical events that make up a larger physiological process. (1.1B: Defining Physiology – Medicine LibreTexts)

Phytonutrient: phytonutrients are nutrients derived from plants.

Quantum Physics: a branch of physics that connects science, psychology, and spirituality and demonstrates that the world and our role in it is malleable to human choice and awareness.

ROI: return on investment.

Self-Directed Neuroplasticity: Dr.Jeffrey M. Schwartz, author of 'The Mind & The Brain', research suggests that the individual plays an active role in influencing neural activity by consciously choosing where to place his or her attention. Before changing habits, it's wise to go upstream and first find a better feeling thought to direct the action you would like to change.

Small Intestinal Bacterial Overgrowth (SIBO): a condition where bacteria from the large intestine migrate their way up into the small intestine. The small intestine is actually supposed to be sterile, but when these bacteria migrate and produce gas, either hydrogen or methane, this leads to abdominal pain. Methane gas causes abdominal distension, bloating, constipation, and pain (it literally temporarily paralyzes portions of the gut). Hydrogen gas tends to cause diarrhea.

SNP: a single nucleotide polymorphism or variant is a change in your DNA code that has the potential to have a profound impact on your health.

Sympathetic Nervous System: the sympathetic nervous system activates the fight or flight response during a threat or perceived danger. It is the division of the nervous system that functions to produce localized adjustments (such as sweating as a response to an increase in temperature) and reflex adjustments of the cardiovascular system.

Symptoms/Illnesses: signs of an underlying imbalance in the systems that keeps your body functioning.

Triggers: are factors that provoke the symptoms and signs of illness.

Vagus Nerve: the tenth cranial nerve also known as the vagal nerve, is the main nerve of your parasympathetic nervous system. This system controls specific body functions such as digestion, heart rate, and immune system.

VCS Test: visual contrast sensitivity testing measures your ability to see details at low contrast levels and is often used as a nonspecific test of neurological function.

Vector-Borne Illness: a disease that results from an infection transmitted to humans and other animals by blood-feeding arthropods, such as ticks, mosquitoes, fleas, bed bugs, lice, sandflies, filth flies, midges, snails, and dust mites, to name several.

H4H CIRS Starter Kit

Hope for Healing (H4H), a pediatric and family practice located in Texas, offers Current Good Manufacturing Practices (cGMP) third-party tested supplements. Third-party testing means anonymous evaluation of the contents of a supplement to determine purity and potency.

To purchase supplements, call Hope for Healing at 281.725.6767 or email hope@get2theroot.com.

This does not replace medical guidance. This is for educational purposes and does not establish a doctor-patient relationship. If you know that your home has been water-damaged, you can decrease the inflammation in your body and "mop up" mycotoxins beginning with the protocol below.

We realize you or your child may be experiencing unbearable pain (showing up as tantrums, tics, and terrifying behaviors) that make it difficult to live life, while you are waiting to become a new patient.

Consider starting with the following suggestions:

- **PEA (Palmitoylethanolamide)—by Neurobiologix:** This a powerful immune modulator of the endocannabinoid system. It is one biochemical step away from anandamide, made within our body. When someone has profound inflammation, you need a *lot* of PEA to support anandamide production. PEA decreases circulating cytokines, relieving literal physical pain but more importantly, decreasing *brain* inflammation/pain.

  - **Children:** If your child cannot swallow capsules, purchase our office's WHITE PEA that does not contain Resveratrol. This capsule is opened up and mixed with food. In general, for children, you can give anywhere from half to one capsule opened up into food twice a day. PEA does not dissolve in liquid. This formula PEA is not directly available from Neurobiolgix.com but was formulated specifically for Hope for Healing. You can safely give the contents of 2 capsules three times a day for 3 weeks for children up to eight years of age when suffering from severe anxiety, then go down to 1 capsule twice a day thereafter.

  - **Adults:** Purchase PEA with Resveratrol. You can take up to three capsules by mouth three times a day for three weeks. PEA helps to stop physical and mental pain due to inflammation caused by cytokines in the body. PEA has the ability to decrease obsessive/compulsive and suicidal thoughts within one to two days if taken at a high dose. Decreasing to a lower dose when your thoughts are stabilized, such as one capsule twice daily, is recommended.

- **GI Detox+ —by Biocidin Botanicals:** This has several binders in it that mop up toxins. Take one hour after a meal and one hour after medication/ supplement ingestion up to two times daily.
  - **Children** can take one capsule twice a day.
  - **Adults** can take two capsules twice a day.

Or

- **Standard Process Okra Pepsin E3 (this is an alternative to GI Detox+ by Biocidin Botanicals.)**
  - **Children** take one capsule three times a day.
  - **Adults** take two capsules three times a day.

- **Fish Oil:**
  - **Children** should take 1200 mg of EPA and 900 mg of DHA daily while treating CIRS. The dose may be decreased when the innate immune system is balanced.
  - **Adults** should take 2400 mg of EPA and 1800 mg of DHA daily.

- **ERMI/HERTSMI Test:** These kits are available at Hope for Healing's office. We recommend that you do both. As of this writing, the kit, with the discount from Envirobiomics, is $210.

- **VCS Test:** This test may be completed from approximately six years of age and above. If failed, continue on the binder until the test is passed. https://www.vcstest.com/ Check your result monthly. When the result is "Negative," you may stop a binder. However, a certain percentage of people will pass the VCS but still will not be feeling well.

Hope for Healing, a pediatric practice located in Texas offers third party testing supplements. You can reach the practice by calling 281-725-6767 ext 3.

The information is for informational purposes only, is not a substitute, and does not render medical or psychological advice, opinion, diagnosis, treatment, or cure. The information provided should not be used for diagnosing or treating a health problem or disease. It is not a substitute for professional care. Always seek the advice of your physician or other qualified healthcare providers with any questions you have regarding your medical conditions and treatment options.

The People of the Waterfall
a folklore tale

There once was a village of people who lived at the base of a huge waterfall by a lovely river. Life was good until one day a stranger was washed over the falls and plummeted to the rocky cauldron of foaming water beneath it.

The people were alarmed and immediately sent two of their best swimmers out to rescue the person. With much effort, the person was dragged ashore and the people succeeded in reviving him.

Before long, another stranger was washed over the falls and again a rescue team was sent into the dangerous waters. As they worked on reviving the person, they decided to station a rescue boat and a lifeline by the base of the falls.

As time passed, strangers continued to be washed over the waterfall and rescue efforts increased. Soon a small building was erected with emergency supplies and designated people were constantly on call for more rescues.

The number of strangers being washed over the fall continued to increase. Soon the people constructed a small hospital at the base of the falls and built a fine rescue boat with full-time emergency rescue workers to staff it.

The people were perplexed but continued to respond to the demands of the victims of the waterfall. They built an even bigger hospital and started to build a whole fleet of rescue boats when at long last, someone asked …

"Why don't we go upstream and see why these people are falling in?"

Welcome to Functional Medicine

Functional medicine goes upstream to understand why so many people are falling over the waterfall and into the pool of chronic dis-ease and developmental delays. Functional medicine is not new. In the 1700s, Hippocrates created a holistic medicine based on man, or microcosm, not the disorder. In the early 1900s, 200 years later, allopathic medicine surfaced with the mindset of one drug for one ailment.

Functional medicine is the science of creating health. It is the medicine of *"why."* Functional medicine takes the *entire person* into consideration when designing a personalized care plan.

This includes your **environment (nutrition, lifestyle, mental, emotional, and spiritual), genetics, and medical (addressing core clinical imbalances).**

What makes functional medicine unique is the acknowledgment that health affects our mindset, our emotions, and our spirituality. Likewise, our mindset, emotions, and spirituality affect our health. With this in mind, you can see that the medical piece is one piece to a much more involved comprehensive care and treatment plan.

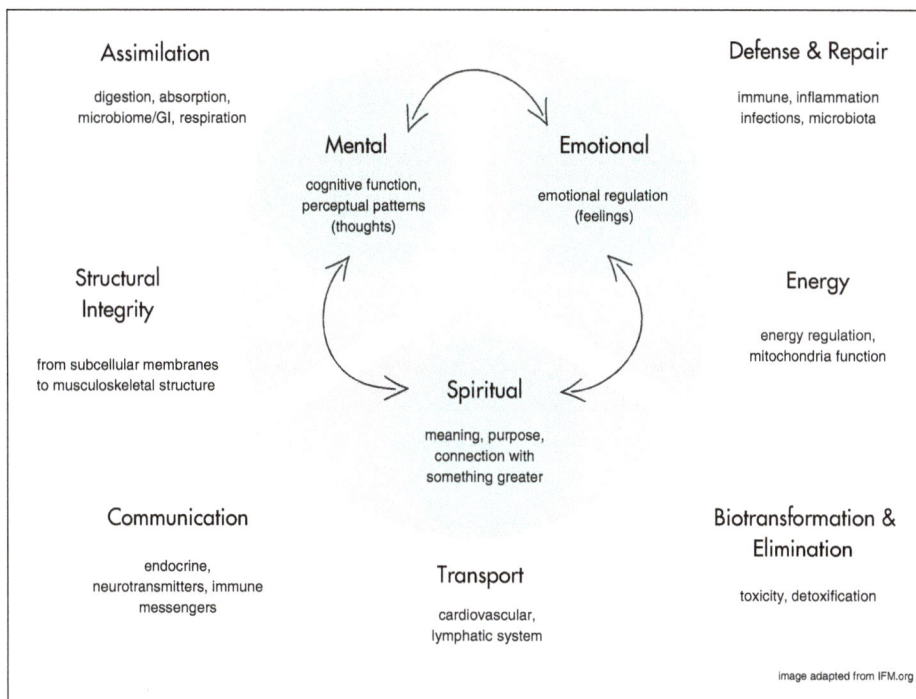

Assimilation
digestion, absorption, microbiome/GI, respiration

Defense & Repair
immune, inflammation infections, microbiota

Mental
cognitive function, perceptual patterns (thoughts)

Emotional
emotional regulation (feelings)

Structural Integrity
from subcellular membranes to musculoskeletal structure

Energy
energy regulation, mitochondria function

Spiritual
meaning, purpose, connection with something greater

Communication
endocrine, neurotransmitters, immune messengers

Transport
cardiovascular, lymphatic system

Biotransformation & Elimination
toxicity, detoxification

image adapted from IFM.org

Principles of
Functional Medicine:

- Focus on a patient-centered, systems-biology approach.
- Evaluation of principal underlying antecedents (family history), triggers (emotional stress, traumatic events, infections), and mediators (ongoing exposures to chemicals, heavy metals, toxins, chronic infections, or stress).
- Mapping your health history timeline to understand how all the influencing factors, over time, have accumulated and interacted with your unique genetic code to express your symptoms of dis-ease.
- In-depth application timing of important dietary, nutraceutical, phytonutrient, mind/body, and pharmacological therapies.
- Detailed clinical applications of core functional laboratory testing.

Functional medicine is a change process. **Each person's change process is different.** Specific experiences and sequence of changes are unique to each individual, however, the nutrition and lifestyle modifications, diagnostic lab testing, supplement protocols, and functional therapies are required for everyone to experience profound results.

This is an exciting time in medicine: doctors and practitioners now understand that even once thought "dead-end diagnoses" can actually be *reversed* by removing the sources of inflammation and repairing the physiological harm from the inflammation that led to disease (such as Alzheimer's disease).

The most common sources of inflammation are

- Emotional stress and trauma
- Dietary (not eating enough, eating too many processed foods, eating too often)
- Gut pathogens (bacteria, fungus, virus, parasites)
- Toxicity (mold, heavy metals, chemicals)
- Financial stress and uncertainty

When the total body burden of inflammation becomes too large, the body responds by expressing symptoms of dis-ease. The sources of inflammation must be removed or greatly reduced/tamed.

Symptoms are
Communication of Deeper
Core Clinical Imbalances

Symptoms are how our body communicates that, somewhere inside us, our body is not performing the right steps in the necessary sequence to maintain health. Once we know where that is happening, and what is causing it, we can begin to learn exactly what to do about it.

Symptoms manifest differently in each patient: headaches, allergies, swollen joints, fatigue, belly pain, constipation, diarrhea, mood swings, rage, irritability, depression, anxiety, pain, thyroid dysfunction, behavioral abnormalities, tics, head-banging, and irritated skin are all symptoms we know well.

Despite spending more than twice what most other industrialized nations spend on healthcare, the US ranks twenty-fourth out of thirty in such nations, in terms of life expectancy. A major reason for this startling fact is we only spend 3 percent of our healthcare dollars on *preventing* diseases.

In the past two decades, we have learned that many of the root causes of the above common symptoms are:

- Emotional, spiritual, and religious stress and trauma
- Physical trauma (injuries and abuse, including sexual abuse)
- Psychological stressors and trauma (abuse, veterans, active-duty military, divorce)
- Biotoxin illness (CIRS)
- Vector-borne illness
- High inflammatory and processed foods
- Finances
- Single Nucleotide Polymorphisms (SNPs)
- Gut dysbiosis (Leaky Gut)
- Immune dysfunction
- Infections (bacterial, viral, fungi, and parasitic overgrowth)
- Mineral and vitamin depletion
- Toxicity (chemicals, heavy metals, biological toxins)
- Root canals and amalgams

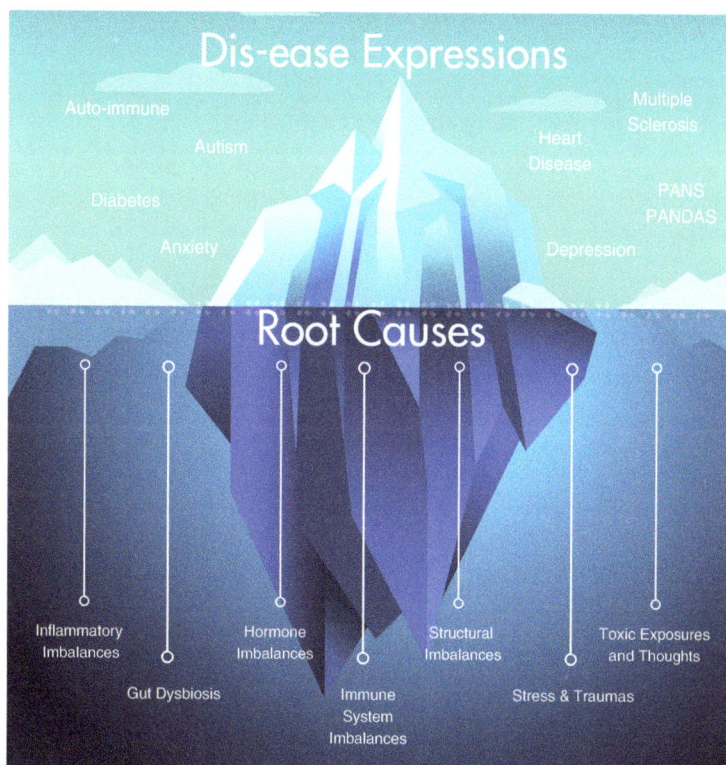

Functional medicine requires that you courageously look at the environment in which you live, including the habitual patterns, which have been created to cope with your environment and unresolved trauma. Habitual patterns include toxic thought patterns, which affect the relationship you have with yourself, your partner, your family, your work, your finances, and your world! Up until now, your environment has been shaping you. *Now is the time when you deliberately and positively affect your environment and claim your health and freedom.*

Functional medicine is participatory medicine, where patients and the collaborative care team work as equal therapeutic partners. **In essence, functional medicine is a process (journey) and a partnership.**

Creating Therapeutic Partnerships

Conventional medicine has taught us that there is something *outside of us* that will make us well again. Many people who seek out functional medicine are still in the mindset that something or someone will *fix them* by doing something for them.

Functional medicine is a mutual-participatory medical model. Therefore, it has shifted the care paradigm from the conventional prescribe-and-treat medical model to empowering the patient/parents to *co-create* their personalized, comprehensive, and coordinated care plan with their medical team as an equal therapeutic partner. Functional medicine positions you as the hero in your story. You are responsible for your unique change process. The medical provider and other collaborative care team members are your guides. The foundation of this curriculum is *to prepare you to assume autonomy in your healthcare to become an effective partner*.

"Tell me and I forget. Teach me and I remember. Involve me and I learn."
Benjamin Franklin

> In order to experience profound results, priority must be placed on removing sources of inflammation with nutrition and lifestyle modifications. Nutrition and lifestyle changes are what establish the foundation upon which all other functional interventions and therapies will be built.

As the patient or parent, you are responsible for designing comprehensive care plans that match your current ability, layer interventions to work in combination, implementing and sustaining the nutrition and lifestyle changes, and medical and therapeutic interventions into your unique and current circumstances. Plus, understanding medical costs and driving well-informed healthcare decisions. Functional medicine's success largely depends on how well a patient or parent can continuously peel back layers of emotional, mental, nutritional, and lifestyle inflammation and sustain those changes.

Your provider is responsible for investigating sources of inflammation with functional diagnostic labs, lab interpretation, personalized supplement, and prescription protocol design, recommending well-timed functional therapies, and nutrition and lifestyle guidance. Your collaborative care team will offer you a strategy to guide you to do this safely, intelligently, and slowly.

Rather than leaving an appointment and cherry-picking what you will actually do, partner with your provider to make a reasonable treatment plan that matches your current ability. **This means you have a voice in the design of your treatment plan.** Being an effective partner means being on the same team. This workbook takes you through discovering your change process to successfully implement and sustain your evolving treatment plans for root cause resolution and symptom remission.

It is our belief that suffering, and challenges reveal our greatest strengths. Much of our growth comes from experiences on that uncomfortable edge where growth really happens. Chronic conditions have the potential to be a catalyst for great change. As a result of learning the lessons that chronic conditions teach, it is common for patients to experience more fulfillment, happiness, and contentment as they move toward health and well-being.

"Change and growth take place when a person has risked himself and dares to become involved with experimenting with his own life." Herbert Otto

The more you are prepared to partner with your care team and to take ownership of your healing journey, to take responsibility for your mindset, emotions, nutrition, and lifestyle, understand medical costs and drive well-informed healthcare decisions with your care team, the more you will benefit from your functional medicine investment.

> **Bottom Line:** Creating comprehensive and coordinated care plans that match your current ability and create consistency and continuity of care is up to you. No medical provider or therapist can do this for you.

Your Functional Medicine Investment Portfolio

We have accepted the social custom of investing in orthodontics, college funds, retirement funds, and investment portfolios. How are you investing income toward your health? You likely purchased this workbook because the path of insurance-covered services is falling short.

Functional medicine is an out-of-pocket investment. And since removing the sources of inflammation, repairing physiological harm, and healing emotional traumas is a process (journey) that takes time, we must think of functional medicine as a portfolio. **Wise investors are committed to long-term gains rather than short-term wins.**

Before you jump into the functional medicine process and partnership, evaluating where you are currently investing your *time* and *money* is wise. These two factors influence the other required nutrition and lifestyle modifications. In Chapter Three, you will work on the new modifiable lifestyle factors: time and money.

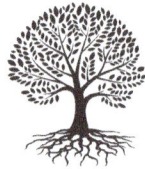

Functional Medicine

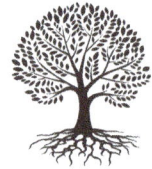

what it is	what it is not
Personalized each individual is unique, and so are their treatments	**Short-term** temporary relief is no one's friend
Identifying Root Causes we dive deep to discover the origins of illness	**Masking Symptoms** prescription drugs can dull the pain but do not heal the root causes
Natural the body has an incredible power to heal if sources of inflammation are removed and it's receiving the proper nutrients	**Quick Fix** it takes time for a flower to blossom, same with your body
Comprehensive optimal well-being is multi-factorial. We leave no stone unturned	**Conventional** treating diseases the same way today as more than 10 years ago
Cutting Edge 21st century approach to medicine	
✅	❌

How to Turn the Initial Boost of Enthusiasm into Endurance for the Journey of Transformation

You've decided to use a functional medicine approach to get back the energy to live life, fit back into your favorite jeans, reverse childhood epidemics like Autism, ease your pain, reverse your chronic disease, sharpen your mind, and lift the cloud of fog over your brain, or simply be proactive about your health and live an optimally healthy, vibrant life. Regardless, *you are unwilling to learn to **manage** your symptoms any longer!* You want to understand what is causing your symptoms!

You're probably feeling excited ... And maybe a little overwhelmed and unprepared? *You are not alone!*

It's easy to get completely overwhelmed, by not only the amount of information available, but also by the out-of-pocket medical expenses, implementing medical protocols, and the number of nutrition and lifestyle changes that need to be made. And you may have tried nutrition and lifestyle changes in the past that didn't seem to make a difference ... or just weren't sustainable for the long term.

It's common to attempt nutrition and lifestyle changes, only for them to quickly feel impossible and unrealistic to maintain. In a short period of time, you can go from an "excited-to-get-started" feeling to feeling like you have very little chance of succeeding.

I want to reassure you: this is normal!

Functional medicine *can* feel overly complex and impossible to maintain, but it doesn't *have* to be this way. In fact, feeling overwhelmed or demoralized is actually just a sign you're doing **too much, too soon for your current ability level.**

If "failures" with nutrition and lifestyle changes and exercise in the past are holding you back from even starting ... I've got good news about that too! **Genetics anyone?**

In truth, there is so much *you can do* to make your journey affordable, sustainable, and successful. The secret is simply knowing where to start and how to sustain your journey ... and that's where health coaching and this workbook comes into play.

This workbook provides you with a structure to discover your own method to design a personalized plan, the confidence and competence to implement your plan into your unique and current circumstances, and most importantly, the knowledge of how to sustain your plan!

No one nutrition or lifestyle modification, supplement, or medical intervention in and of itself will resolve all your pains. It's an accumulation of all pieces to a comprehensive care plan, including the mental, emotional, and spiritual components, working in combination that will create the results (gains) you desire. *So much positive change can happen in one year's time.*

"*Simplicity is what will convert the initial boost of enthusiasm into endurance for the long journey.*" Kara Ware

The Role of the Health Coach

Assisting You in Designing *Your* Method to Navigate Your Functional Medicine Journey

In addition to your medical providers, another important partner in the functional medicine model is a health coach. The coach knows this path well and assists you through your change process. As you, the hero in your own story, venture into a different way of thinking, talking, and behaving, it's helpful to have a seasoned guide walk alongside you.

The coach is your ally; the person who walks next to you as you climb your mountain. The coach knows the mountain well, and helps you plan your climb. Together, you assess your big vision, your desires, and your readiness for the climb, and examine what you have and what you need in mindset, equipment, and resources. Together a route is determined.

The coach cannot make you climb but rather works with you to find your motivation and strengths required to journey through the peaks and valleys.

The coach is there with you to help encourage you through the temptation to turn back prematurely (as you may have done in the past). As we know, change isn't easy, or we would all be radiantly healthy!

This workbook provides a structure for you to discover your method to be well prepared to partner with your care team and feel confident and competent to live your personalized plan—**you become the solution.**

The Curriculum "At a glance"

Chapter One: Designing Your Plan: Create your personalized, comprehensive, and coordinated nutrition and lifestyle plan

Chapter Two: Implementing Your Plan: Emotional | Mental | Spiritual

Chapter Three: Sustaining Your Plan: Time | Finances | Nonviolent communication

Chapter Four: Telling Your Story: Prepare for your partnership and inspire others

Goals: The cornerstone of functional medicine is empowerment. The conventional prescribe-and-treat model removes autonomy over your healthcare decisions. This workbook aims to empower you to be an equal, therapeutic partner with your providers. As an equal partner, you are responsible for implementing the modifiable lifestyle changes, which allows the medical interventions to provide the profound results we all know are possible with root-cause healing. You are writing your story of hope and healing.

Understandings: Functional medicine is a mutual-participatory medical model. How well a patient or parent can implement the nutrition and lifestyle changes drives the needle in functional medicine. 80 percent of functional medicine is lifestyle medicine. Modifiable lifestyle factors are the foundation all other functional medicine interventions will build upon. Functional medicine is only successful when you fulfill your role as a partner in your healthcare; no one intervention or no one person can "fix" you or your child. Healing is much more than taking supplements and changing what you eat. The mental, emotional, and spiritual healing is where you have the most power to influence your outcome.

Skills: You will understand the influencing factors which have accumulated over time to burden your biological and neurological systems and create your unique symptom set. You will identify sources of inflammation that are initiators of illness. You will be competent in designing your nutrition and lifestyle plan that matches your current ability. Every three months, you will update your nutrition and lifestyle plan and layer on more changes to work in combination. This is the layering method that you will master. You will know your values, strengths, and sources of inspiration to develop a functional mindset to implement your chosen changes successfully. Plus, you will budget your time and money and improve your communication skills to sustain your path of transformation.

Self-Assessments: Your workbook and care planner are partnership tools to design, organize, implement, document, track, budget, and sustain your three-month plans to best partner with your family, medical professionals, and therapists. Your partnership tools will document where you are starting, what you are willing to do, the time and money you invest in creating a reasonable, livable plan, and track your symptoms and changes. Food Journals, the MSQ (Medical Symptom Questionnaire), Promis10, and Positive Intelligence PQ score assessment tools are recommended tracking tools to chart progress. We recommend taking these assessments every 90 days. **Parents:** we recommend you take these assessments for yourself and not your child. This is as much your healing journey as it is your child's.

Learning Outcomes:

- Understand your timeline: understand how your family history (antecedents), stress, trauma, and infections (triggers), and ongoing exposures (mediators) have accumulated and have resulted in the expression of your unique symptom set. You must first understand why you have tipped into certain disease states to determine the path toward root-cause resolution.

- Design a nutrition and lifestyle plan that matches your current ability (current ability = motivation + competence + confidence).

- Discover the emotional, mental, and spiritual skills to implement your personalized, comprehensive, and coordinated care plan.

- Create a mindset that transforms your greatest challenge into your greatest teacher to become the best, most courageous version of yourself.

- Identify potential roadblocks and what you will rely on in times of increased chaos, stress, and adversity.
- Plan realistic goals to reduce challenges, frustrations, and overwhelm.
- Transform sabotaging expectations.
- Learn communication and interpersonal skills to go against the cultural norm, build better relationships, and sustain your functional medicine journey.
- Budget your time and money to invest wisely.
- Establish a strong foundation for future medical interventions to be successful.

The Power in Preparing

Start here

First, look for self-acceptance. It is easy to see everything that your symptoms have negatively impacted. It is not as easy to look at what you are gaining from your journey when you are in the darkest hours. Accept that you are right where you are supposed to be, doing exactly what you should be doing. *Accepting the challenges in front of you and learning to influence them with love and patience* is a main theme throughout this workbook.

> *"Every adversity, every failure, every heartbreak carries with it the seed of an equal or greater benefit."* Napoleon Hill.

Second, begin to document your family history, triggering and traumatic life events, and ongoing exposures such as processed food intake, mold/bacterial toxin exposures, tick bites, heavy metal exposures, dental fillings (amalgams), etcetera. Functional medicine is a search for the root cause of symptoms. To do this, we need to understand the sources of inflammation. **It is imperative to understand the past to inform the future.** This helps not only prepare you for your medical visit but the more thorough timeline you provide to your medical provider with approximate dates of the events better prepares your provider to formulate your medical plan. Functional medicine is all about an inflammation hunt. Understanding that your or your child's symptoms did not appear overnight or out of nowhere but are an accumulation of inflammatory exposures is **key** to setting reasonable expectations when creating your short- and long-term goals.

Transforming any instant gratification expectation to an agreement that functional medicine is a process (journey), and a partnership is essential to your success. **This is not a quick fix! However, small steps add up to big changes. A lot of positive change can occur in one year.**

The third step is to write a food journal. Write everything you and your child eat for four days without judgment. This is simply taking inventory of where you are on your functional medicine journey. Complete food journals every three months to track your progress.

And fourth, take the VIA Character Strengths Assessment. The VIA survey at viacharacter.org provides insight into your top character strengths. Note that everyone possesses strengths, and all are good. The survey lists the strengths of those you use the most and descending to the least. This is in preparation for Chapter Two. Learning to rely on your strengths is pivotal to designing, implementing, and sustaining your transformation journey. Also, consider taking the Positive Intelligence PQ score assessment. The PQ Score is the indicator for the percentage of time your mind is acting like your friend, instead of your enemy. https://www.positiveintelligence.com/saboteurs/

"The real tragedy of life is not that each of us doesn't have enough strengths; it's that we fail to use the ones we have." Marcus Buckingham and Donald O. Clifton

Chapter 1: Designing Your Plan

Key Terms

Mutual-Participatory Medical Model: different from the prescribe and treat model, the mutual-participatory medical model is where patient and provider work together as equal partners to co-create a reasonable and evolving care plan.

Layering Method: layering pieces of a comprehensive care plan to work together in combination.

Stabilization: before evolving your care plan, stabilize your plan by not making any additional changes for at least 2-weeks. A period to stabilize changes allows the interventions to integrate and become part of your consistent lifestyle.

3-month care plans: 90-days gives enough time to implement changes, stabilize the changes, and then evolve your plan for the next 3 months.

5Rs- Remove, Replace, Reinoculate, Repair, and Rebalance.

High-Allergen Foods: gluten, dairy, corn, and soy are the big 4 to remove.

Nutrigenomics: uncovers the relationship between an individual's

genes, nutrition, and wellness.

SNPs: (single nucleotide polymorphisms) SNPs are slight variations that are actually what makes you unique.

Current Ability: changes you have sufficient motivation, confidence, and competence to implement successfully.

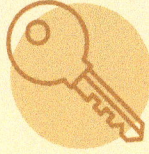

Learning Outcomes

Part 1: Creating a Personalized Nutrition and Lifestyle Plan Based on Your Current Ability

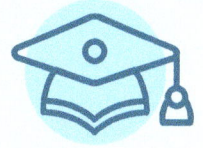

- What is functional medicine?
- Acknowledging the roles and responsibilities of the patient, provider, and care team.
- Realizing overwhelm is a sign you are doing too much, too fast.
- Mapping your timeline.
- Evaluating sources of inflammation.
- Removing high allergen foods.
- Be familiar with modifiable change domains.
- Identify your values and character strengths.
- Design your 90-day nutrition and lifestyle plan based on your current ability.
- Using the Menu of Nutrition and Lifestyle Options section.
- Discovering the Layering Method.
- Planning for periods of stabilization.
- Introduction to nutrigenomics.
- Selecting supplements based on purity and potency.

Part 2: The Stages of Change.

- Acknowledging there are more stages than action in the change process.
- Using the Stages of Change to customize your personalized plan.
- Acknowledging *no one intervention alone will solve all pains*. Removing x and expecting y to happen is not how it works.

Part 1: Creating a Personalized Lifestyle Plan Based on Current Ability

What is Functional Medicine?

The Institute for Functional Medicine defines the functional medicine approach on their website like this:

"Functional medicine is a systems biology–based approach that focuses on identifying and addressing the root cause of disease. Functional medicine determines how and why illness occurs and restores health by addressing the root causes of disease for each individual.

This is a mutually empowering relationship between patient and provider where both share responsibility for creating and implementing the healthcare plan to achieve desired well-being."

Patient-Provider Therapeutic Partnership

By now, you know functional medicine is a mutual-participatory medical model where the patient and provider work as equal therapeutic partners. This is very different from the prescribe-and-treat medical model. Allopathic medicine is wonderful for emergencies, however, the model for treating chronic diseases has become known as sick-care.

Each Partner Has Roles and Responsibilities

The mutual-participatory medical model centers on establishing and working within an equal, therapeutic patient-provider partnership. As the patient or parent, you are responsible for designing your comprehensive and coordinated care plan, learning how to implement and sustain nutrition and lifestyle changes, and incorporating the medical recommendations into your unique and current circumstances. Your provider is responsible for investigating sources of inflammation with functional diagnostic labs, lab interpretation, personalized supplement and prescription protocol design, recommending well-timed functional therapies, and nutrition and lifestyle guidance.

To assist in facilitating the success of the partnership is the Collaborative Care Team. Each care team member is equally valuable and necessary as medical providers. We have already established the role of a health coach. Patient care coordinators, customer service representatives, medical scribes, triage nurses, and medical assistants may all be a part of the care team you inherit. Other collaborative care team partners are behavioral optometrists, bodywork therapists, biological dentists, chiropractors, osteopathic physicians, master herbalists, energy workers, physicians, biomagnetism specialists, and other counseling therapists. We ask that you treat your Collaborative Care Team with respect, kindness, and dignity. Every professional realizes the stress and grief you shoulder and is ready to partner with and guide you to hope and to heal.

Healing complex medical conditions is a big undertaking. It takes time and a team! It might feel overwhelming to look at your whole life, make big nutrition and lifestyle changes, and follow medical protocols. This is why we highly encourage you to include a coach in your team.

Comprehensive and Coordinated Care Plans

Healthcare is fragmented! It is a terrifying maze to navigate. I authored this workbook to walk you through designing, implementing, and sustaining your root cause, personalized care plans to effectively partner with your healthcare providers to experience transformational healing.

When you and/or your child are struggling or in obvious pain, and your or your child's symptoms and behaviors are terrifying, possibly feel unmanageable, or are bothersome, you want to see the doctor immediately. Rightfully so! You or your child need medical oversight! However, the medical piece is just one part of a comprehensive care plan.

Regardless if you are the patient or a parent of a child living with a chronic condition/developmental delay, it's crucial to develop the skill set to design your comprehensive and coordinated care plan that fosters consistency and continuity of care. No medical provider or therapist can connect and layer all the pieces of a comprehensive care plan, implement, and sustain the plan for you. That is your responsibility, and it is challenging considering the abundance of information to sift and sort through and the number of professionals who are part of your care team.

When people seek personalized, functional medicine and invest in a functional medicine provider, they look for what the provider can do *for* them. There is nothing magical your provider can do to resolve all of your or your child's pains. A functional medical provider offers strategy and advanced medical interventions and protocols to address vector-borne illnesses, detoxification of biotoxins, heavy metals, and chemicals, kill gut pathogens like viruses, bacteria, fungi, and parasites, induce cellular autophagy, and regenerate neuronal growth and synaptic connections. But before it's safe to implement another protocol to kill, detoxify, induce, and regenerate, it's intelligent to strengthen everyone's constitution (including parents) by peeling back more mental, emotional, spiritual, nutritional, and lifestyle inflammation.

This workbook is a compilation of research in systems biology medicine, metacognition, positive psychology, narrative therapy, self-directed neuroplasticity, brain-heart coherence, quantum physics, mind-body medicine, nonviolent communication, and time and financial budgeting. The field of behavioral sciences is the implementation vehicle for systems biology medicine called functional medicine.

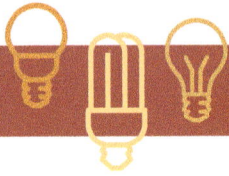

The Comprehension section is intended to optimize your comprehension. This section reviews the big ideas which make functional medicine provide the profound results we have come to expect. Think about what you have learned and how you will apply them to your unique and current circumstances.

What really drives the needle in optimizing clinical outcomes?

What are the roles and responsibilities of the patients and the parents of patients?

Mapping Your Timeline

Before we set off for an adventure, a vacation, or even choose a college, we do some planning. To create a plan that is right for you, it's important first to understand the past. Understanding the past better informs the future. Although young children or newborns do not have as long of a health history as adults, they still have their family health history, pregnancy, delivery, and exposures. Mapping your timeline means to write down the last time you felt well and begin to write down your **Antecedents,** family's health history and what you know about your genetics. Write down the time frames (month/year) for **Triggers** such as traumatic, often sudden events that "trigger" symptoms to appear on the scene, like a car accident, divorce, surgery, infection, sexual/physical abuse, or a potential adverse medication or vaccine reaction. And finally, write down **Mediators,** those ongoing exposures like antibiotics, water-damaged buildings full of mold/bacteria, mercury tooth amalgams, the Standard American Diet (SAD), and exposures to agricultural or industrial chemicals.

Vaccine dates are imperative to include in your timeline.

Disclaimer*
Read the article listed in the Bibliography, the third-leading cause of death in the US that most doctors don't want you to know about.

Sources of Inflammation

Functional medicine is an inflammation hunt. The most common sources of inflammation are:

- Dietary: eating too many processed foods, eating too often, not eating enough
- Mental | Emotional | Physical | Spiritual | Sexual stress and trauma
- Financial stress and uncertainty
- Gut pathogens: bacteria, fungi, viruses, parasites
- Toxicity: bacteria, mold, chemicals, heavy metals

This workbook focuses on the first three sources of inflammation. You and your medical provider will focus on the last two. The basic tenets of functional medicine are the **5Rs: Remove, Replace, Reinoculate, Repair,** and **Rebalance.**

In our experience, most patients begin to experience results with the first two Rs alone because removing sources of inflammation and replacing them with nutrient-dense, whole food, and quality supplements to replace missing vitamins and minerals begin the repair process. Working on the removing and replacing parts of the 5R approach, before you meet your medical provider, allows you to work immediately with your provider on the reinoculating, repairing, and rebalancing phases when you have your initial medical consultation.

Removing, Replacing High-Allergen Foods

By now, you completed a 4-day food journal where you wrote down everything you or your child ate without judgment. You took inventory of where you are currently on your functional medicine journey. It's recommended to repeat the food journaling exercise every three months to track your progress. **Ideally, you will have removed many high inflammatory foods before you meet with your medical provider.**

Be mindful to replace high-allergen foods with whole foods or minimally processed foods with few ingredients. It's common for people to fall into the "gluten-free crap trap." These gluten-free products are still highly processed and by no means healthy foods.

Gluten and dairy are addictive. The food industry knows that, too. So, they package gluten with fat and sugar (from Barley, Rice, Oats, Wheat, and Spelt: BROWS acronym—makes it easy to remember what contains gliadin, the protein in wheat, that causes so many reactions). The food industry gives us "food-like substances" or "Frankenfood," but it doesn't provide our body with nutrients to grow and flourish and think and gain new milestones, like speech, fine and gross motor coordination.

Dairy products contain casein, one of the proteins in milk.

Both gluten and casein form short-chain opioids (yes, narcotics) that cross the blood brain barrier and bind to opioid receptors. Gluten and dairy are a literal addiction. This is one root cause creating picky eating.

Unfortunately, it takes about five days for the sheer desire for dairy and gluten to go away.

Dr. K suggests removing dairy first. Substitute "lateral shifts," like coconut milk that is carrageenan free or possibly a nut milk. (Carrageenan is an inflammatory substance used as a thickening agent made from red and purple algae. Avoid it!) If your child is greater than one year old and less than three years old, use water or coconut milk because they need healthy fat for brain development through 36 months of age. Removing dairy frequently improves eye contact in your child with autism.

Next, remove all the gluten from the house, including gluten cross-reactive foods like corn, millet, rice, and yeast. It's VERY HARD, but it CAN be done!

The Magic Pill (movie: https://www.imdb.com/title/tt6035294/) did a beautiful job showing how moods and personalities change when you remove these dreadful addictive foods that inflame you or your child's brain and instead provide nourishing whole foods.

There are so many resources available today to guide you in replacing high-allergen foods. Keywords to search for are the Elimination Diet, Specific Carbohydrate Diet, modified Paleo (to reduce the amount of saturated fat), and the Mediterranean Diet.

A note for parents: Your child may not eat for three to five days, but then they will eat. Giving real food (poultry, meat, vegetables, fruit) is calming and is possible.

As you replace these addictive foods, your child's behaviors may amplify. Please know this is normal and will pass. It is highly unlikely they will starve themselves. When tantrums are in full swing, whispering to your child is advisable. Let them know that this is not who they are; this is the diagnosis you are healing.

Tell them they are smart, fun, and beautiful and that you love them so much that you will no longer provide them with food that makes them sick with eczema, autism, Crohn's disease, etcetera. After all, you wouldn't feed them any other kind of poison. Change your belief that "a little bit of dairy or gluten won't hurt." **That is not true when reversing serious chronic conditions and developmental delays!** When they are calm, give them lateral shift options to replace their toxic snacks of Cheez-It©, Goldfish© crackers, or chicken nuggets.

Let them know they will start feeling much better and, therefore, will have way more fun. Whisper that they are teaching you to help the entire family feel better. Thank them. Let your eyes shine with love and your breathing and body be calm. This is why you have to train your mind and emotions. This is how you reduce resistance.

If they push away the food you are serving, please be calm and patient. Tell them, *"That's okay; you can eat this later when you are hungry."* Please do not get up and provide them with something else they may like better. Watch out for this tendency, and know they are training you! You must parent your child rather than parenting from a place of fearing the autism, or diagnosis. **You have to decide who is in charge. You or the dis-ease.**

Our children can understand us even if it looks like they are in a far-off galaxy. Reassure them you know what needs to be done and that many people are helping uncover them from the (diagnosis). It's important to teach your children what you are doing and why. You are teaching them to partner with you. As you continue your healing journey, you will be surprised by how much your child learns to work with you on their care plan.

> *"When I first tried to make lateral shifts, my nonverbal son would gag and resist the new foods I tried to introduce. As I became more committed to no longer providing the foods he would eat since they were perpetuating his dis-ease state, he would immediately go into meltdown mode. After a while, I realized there were about four meltdowns before he accepted what I had to offer. With each meltdown, I knew I was getting closer to his acceptance. My son did not eat for seven days. He asked for a sandwich on day four. I didn't even know he knew that word! On the eighth day, he ate baked acorn squash with ghee and has never again balked at his food options."* Kari M, parent.

Values and Strengths

In 1999, Neil Mayerson, PhD was concerned that inadequate progress was being made in psychology from well-worn problem-fixing approaches and that an approach based on recognizing people's strengths and aspirations might prove more effective.

IEP (Individualized Education Plan) meetings, DSM (Diagnostic and Statistical Manual of Mental Disorders), and ICD codes (International Classification of Diseases) describe and measure much of what is wrong with people. Insurance companies and HMOs (Health Maintenance Organizations) reimburse the treatment of disorders but certainly not the correction of root causes or promotion of health, happiness, and fulfillment.

Dr. Mayerson founded the VIA Institute and asked Dr. Martin Seligman, PhD, known as the father of Positive Psychology, to become the scientific director. He asked Christopher Peterson, PhD to be its project director. This was a turning point in psychology and really for medicine. Until then, the field primarily focused on what was wrong with a person and what needed fixing.

In essence, Mayerson asked, *"How else can we view a person other than through their neurosis and pathologies?"* He wanted to know about those things that are right with an individual, specifically about the strengths of character that make the good life possible. This is the basis of positive psychology, and this question initiated thirty years of behavioral science research substantiating how change happens.

Mayerson says studies have shown that when people focused on strengths, they were more successful. When people who initially focused on their weaknesses began to focus on their strengths, they became more successful.

You are much more than a collection of symptoms. I encourage you to dig deep and identify your values. Connect every thought you think, word you speak, and action you take to your values rather than your dis-ease. Your journey is *"transforming your personality to create a new personal reality,"* and this is done by building upon what you are already doing well and looking for more ways to feel good. When the changes you are making feel good, you will naturally look for what more **you can do.** The goal is *not* to keep your life as much like it was before the illness occurred but rather allow this journey to change you for the better. Learn more about placing your values into action with character strengths at viacharacter.org.

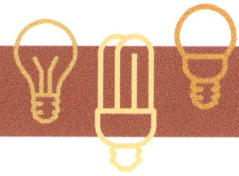

The Comprehension section is intended to optimize your comprehension. This section reviews the big ideas which make functional medicine provide the profound results we have come to expect. Think about what you have learned and how you will apply them to your unique and current circumstances.

I understand the five main sources of inflammation are

When I think about my sources, or my child's sources of inflammation, I think of...

Modifiable Lifestyle Changes

80 percent of a functional medicine plan is modifying your nutrition and lifestyle; 20 percent is implementing your provider's well-timed medical interventions.

You can take a multitude of nutritional and anti-inflammatory supplements and invest in diagnostic labs and functional therapies (exosomes, stem cells, IV therapy, etcetera), but if you are <u>not</u> *eating anti-inflammatory foods and living a lifestyle* that positively affects your biological symptoms, your symptoms will remain.

By first establishing a foundation with the required nutrition and lifestyle changes, this will allow the medical interventions to be successful. This is what we refer to as an intelligent sequence.

By placing priority on the basics (the modifiable lifestyle factors), **you** can expedite your or your child's healing process. Toward the end of this workbook, you will find a Menu of Nutrition and Lifestyle Options. The menu of options is a summary of all *you can do* to remove sources of inflammation contributing to the symptoms you are experiencing.

The functional medicine modifiable lifestyle domains are

- Stress and Resilience Modifications
- Nutrition Modifications
- Lifestyle & Environment Modifications
- Sleep & Relaxation Modifications
- Movement & Exercise Modifications
- Relationship Modifications
- Time and Money Modifications

A note for parents: At the very beginning of your workbook, we introduced the philosophy that this functional medicine journey is something you do **with** your children, not something you **do to** them. This is not another therapy that focuses solely on the child. If you attempt to change your child's nutrition without changing you or the entire family, you are setting yourself up for more tantrums and resistance. We recommend you create your three-month **Family Care Plan**. Your child's health challenges are guiding you to embark on your own healing journey. You are 100 percent in control of what comes into your house. In Chapter 4, we introduce the concept to make your home a safe zone. If you would like help with parenting skills to communicate with all of your children about the changes, please email us and we will either provide parenting support and/or connect you with a parenting coach.

And regarding your other children, it's equally as important to teach them what you are doing and why. You are teaching them how to protect their health as they grow into adults. Siblings can still eat their favorite foods outside of the home and with friends, but the desire is to move everyone to healthier choices at all times.

Build Your Personalized Care Plan

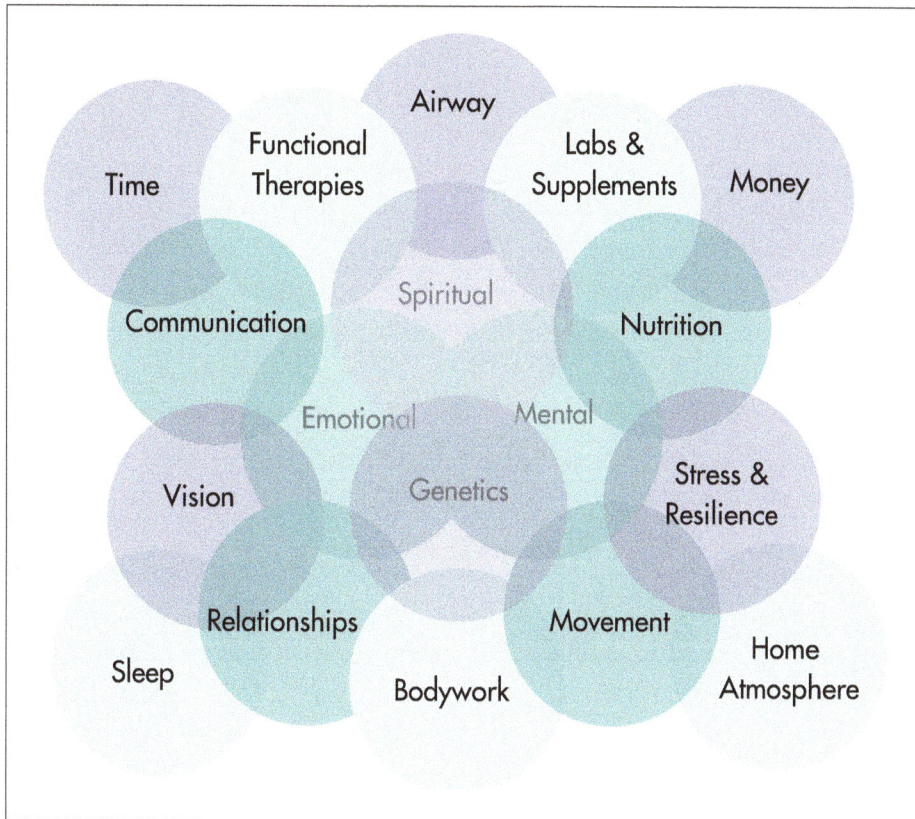

Airway
Functional Therapies
Labs & Supplements
Time
Money
Spiritual
Communication
Nutrition
Emotional
Mental
Vision
Genetics
Stress & Resilience
Relationships
Movement
Sleep
Bodywork
Home Atmosphere

No one medical intervention, supplement, nutrition, or lifestyle change will in and of itself resolve all your pains. Instead, layering many pieces of a comprehensive care plan to work together over time is what eventually restores your or your child's well-being and freedom. The medical piece is just one piece of a comprehensive care plan.

A comprehensive care plan can include but is not limited to removing high-allergen foods, relationships/support, hydration, stress & resilience, sleep, movement, home atmosphere, time and money management, nonviolent communication, airway, vision, functional therapies, labs, supplements, pharmaceuticals, structural integration and bodywork, genetics, plus the individual's mental, emotional, and spiritual aspects of health and well-being.

We can't do everything all at once, and there is an intelligent sequence of layering interventions. Our team works with you to prioritize and design a personalized care plan that prepares you for more advanced medical interventions and, most importantly, a plan you feel good about implementing and sustaining. After each encounter, we want you to feel like "Yes! I can do this!" If that's not the feeling, your collaborative care team needs to know so you walk out the door with a plan that matches your current ability. This is the method for preventing a financial, emotional, and healing crisis.

In the back of your workbook, you will find a Menu of Nutrition and Lifestyle Changes. Choose changes that feel good to you, and those that you feel are reasonable to accomplish in 90-days. Each day, think, "What is just one thing I can do right now for my 90-day care plan?" Keep it simple! If you think that thought throughout the day, you will be successful. By shifting your focus to each moment, you may achieve more tremendous success than anything you could have imagined!

*It's advisable to choose changes you and your partner can agree upon.

Every three months, update your care plan by choosing the next nutrition and lifestyle changes that match your current motivation, competence, and confidence (current ability). Your medical provider will update your medical protocols. Once you add a change to your plan, maintain it. This is called the **Layering Method**. The changes that may have initially felt impossible will soon enough become possible. It's highly recommended that you continuously become more devoted to mastering nutrition and lifestyle changes. As you continue your journey, you will layer more changes to work in combination with the previous three-month plan.

Working in 90-day increments allows change and stabilization to occur. Three-month increments will enable you to experience short-term wins that build momentum toward actualizing your long-term vision. **Planning for stabilization is the most *overlooked* component of a successful and sustainable care plan.** You are eager to get over your own or your child's symptoms, so you may keep trying to do as much as you can as quickly as possible—which keeps your body locked in that fight-or-flight sympathetic nervous system. Being on this "hamster wheel" can send you into a healing crisis. In order to rest and digest (parasympathetic mode), you must include times of stabilization to allow the interventions to integrate and become part of your consistent lifestyle before layering in the next set of nutrition and lifestyle changes. It's highly recommended that at the end of 90-days, you take at least two weeks to not add anything new. This is the perfect time to begin creating your next 90-day plan while you stabilize the changes you have put into motion.

And most importantly, place priority on the person you are becoming rather than your end-desired outcome. Small steps add up over time to create significant change! A lot of positive change can happen in one year!

> *"A plan is bringing the future into the present so you can do something about it."* Alan Lakein

"Simplicity changes behavior." Dr. BJ Fogg

Most people think to heal the underlying causes creating their symptoms, they need to do something radical—go big or go home—which, honestly, is the recipe for self-criticism and disappointment and the exact reason why people start functional medicine and then quickly feel like they can't do all of this, and chalk up functional medicine as something they tried that did not work. Adapting and sustaining mental, emotional, nutritional, and lifestyle changes can feel hard, and people find themselves unable to correct the course. Since transformative healing outcomes heavily rely on how well a patient or parent can implement and sustain modifiable lifestyle changes, viewing nutrition and lifestyle changes as skill development is essential. The key is to build self-efficacy, the feeling *you can* change.

Dr. BJ Fogg wrote the book *Tiny Habits: The Small Changes That Change Everything.* Fogg provides an evidence-based behavior change model that helps you select, design, and implement simple, healthy habits that become routine.

According to Fogg, habits grow by helping people do what they already want to do and helping people feel successful. To do this, Fogg teaches three universal elements of behavior change: **M**otivation, **A**bility, and **P**rompt. A behavior change happens when the three elements of MAP come together at the exact moment, B=MAP.

Fogg defines **M**otivation as behavior the patient wants to do. This is how he recommends helping people do what they already want to do. Interestingly, Fogg points out that Motivation waxes and wanes; it fluctuates. He calls attention to the fact that it is normal for people to experience bursts of motivation, and then life gets hard, and the motivation busts, and people feel demoralized and doubtful they can change and heal. Fogg also points out there are many competing motivators, like I want to rest *and* I want to work out, making people ambivalent about changing. Fogg says motivation is unreliable, so it is not enough alone to drive change. He explains that people can only achieve aspirations and outcomes (life goals) when people execute the *right specific behaviors.*

People start with high motivation and often choose behavior changes outside their current ability. I observe patients and parents choosing to address their most ingrained habits first, ultimately leaving them feeling like they don't have enough willpower. It is essential to notice willpower is not a universal element of change.

Ability is where people have the **most power** to influence their behavior changes. Motivation will vary, but *ability will improve*, thus increasing confidence—fueling self-efficacy. If you want to make a habit consistent, you've got to adjust the most reliable thing in Fogg's B=MAP behavior change model ... Ability. Fogg teaches the Ability Chain and the importance of identifying weak links in your perceived current ability. Fogg's Ability Chain includes five factors: time, money, physical effort, mental effort, and routine. Fogg's Discovery Question, "What is making this behavior hard to do?" narrows down which ability chain factor needs to be supported.

Do you have enough **time?**

Do you have enough **money?**

Are you **physically capable** of doing the behavior?

Does the behavior require a lot of creative or **mental energy?**

Does the behavior fit into your **current routine,** or does it require you to make adjustments?

To improve ability and make behavior change feel easier, ask Fogg's breakthrough question, *"How can I make this behavior easier?"* To make a behavior change feel easier, Fogg suggests looking for tools, resources, and scaling back the behavior to manipulate the ability element to work in your favor. Working within ability (tiny behaviors) is a good indicator of what habits are more or less likely to become habits. Incremental progress that leads to sustainable success is not the priority in most people's minds. Small is not sexy, but it is successful and sustainable. Fogg says, *"When it comes to changing habits, the solution is to make it ridiculously easy to do. Keeping behaviors tiny allows the new habit to root into routine."*

P is for a prompt. A prompt is defined as a cue to do the specific behavior; prompts remind us to act; it says, do this now. No behavior change happens without a prompt—no prompt, no behavior change.

Matching oneself with the right specific behaviors is the most critical step in Fogg's behavior design process and an important place to return when troubleshooting. Behavior matching is selecting the right specific behaviors from the swarm of possible behavior changes that match the person's motivation and ability and choosing the changes that will have the most impact. This is Fogg's systematic criteria for selecting the right specific behaviors to help you answer... *"How can I do this?"*

Choosing behaviors that set one up for success increases confidence and mastery as you go, thus increasing your natural motivation to do bigger and bigger behaviors. Fogg calls this laddering up. He says, *"Understanding the machinery of human behavior—we can deconstruct efforts at changes and how they are being undermined or supported."*

The power of feeling good is the best way to create habits. There is a direct connection between what you feel when you do behavior and the likelihood that you will repeat the behavior in the future. Remember, we need behavior change persistence! *"Positive emotions are habit fertilizer."* says Fogg. Celebrations are the best way to create a positive feeling that wires in your new habits. A celebration is something you do to create a positive feeling inside of yourself. Something simple, like clapping three times after you accomplish your tiny habit. Fogg finds that people can form habits very quickly, often in just a few days, as long as people have strong positive emotions connected to the behavior. Fogg wants you to celebrate tiny successes. He says, *"Celebration will one day be ranked alongside mindfulness and gratitude as a daily practice that contributes most to our overall happiness and well-being."*

To get the cliff notes on Fogg's behavior change model, visit autismremission.com and download my free Foundations First Behavior Change PDF.

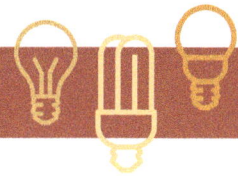

The Comprehension section is intended to optimize your comprehension. This section reviews the big ideas which make functional medicine provide the profound results we have come to expect. Think about what you have learned and how you will apply them to your unique and current circumstances.

I've already removed the following sources of inflammation

A few things that have been going well in my healing journey are

The next modifiable changes I'm interested in learning more about are

I feel motivated to layer in these next changes that are a match to my current competency and confidence

In 90-days I hope to accomplish

To help me make these changes, I'm relying on

Research the Elimination Diet. It's called the Elimination Diet because it's helping you eliminate your symptoms!

Adding in Supplements to Your Care Plan

Supplementing with nutrients is a big piece of a functional medicine care plan. Therefore, it is important to understand a few key considerations.

Potency and Purity of Supplements

Your medical provider has vetted third-party tested brands, free from high allergens and common contaminants, and have the levels of potency that he/she relies on, just like medications. **Supplements are not FDA regulated**. Purchasing supplements at grocery stores or convenience store markets is not advisable because supplements from grocery stores are typically **food grade.**

The third-party tested supplements will be more expensive than what you can find at a grocery store or large retail store. Since supplements are not regulated, fillers and toxins are common in less reputable brands. We highly encourage you to follow your provider's recommendations and purchase high-quality supplement brands.

Supplements alone **will not** heal the underlying causes creating your symptoms; the supplements will be a wise investment when working in tandem with nutrition and lifestyle changes. You must have noninflammatory, nourishing foods in place before you attempt to supplement with other nutrients ... after all, supplements are added to a diet of whole, real foods.

We need to banish the one pill for one ailment belief. Although certain supplements address nutrient deficiencies, toxins, or gut pathogens, remember the additional nutrients are supporting the entire body, plus the mind, emotions, and spiritual components that move you toward well-being. Please do not expect to take one supplement to heal one symptom.

Here are a few supplement starter kits Dr. K recommends while you wait to see your medical provider.

To purchase supplements, call Hope for Healing or email hope@get2theroot.com.

We highly recommend that you start with one supplement at a time and slowly layer each one in, spacing each supplement out by 3-7 days. If you see an increase in negative symptoms, lower the dose/frequency, and see if the symptoms dissipate. Remember to document these adjustments in your Personalized Care Planner.

Hope for Healing (H4H): Supplement Starter Kits

H4H Beginning Autism Kit
(while you are waiting for your genetics and medical consult):

PEA Soothe Support (WHITE):
- **Children:** If your child cannot swallow capsules, purchase the WHITE PEA that does not contain Resveratrol from our office. This capsule is opened up and

mixed with food. In general, for children, you can give anywhere from half to one capsule opened up into food twice a day. PEA does not dissolve in liquid. This formula PEA is not directly available from Neurobiolgix.com but was formulated specifically for Hope for Healing. You can safely give the contents of 2 capsules three times a day for 3 weeks for children up to 8 years of age when suffering from severe anxiety, then go down to 1 capsule twice a day thereafter.

- **Adults:** purchase the PEA with Resveratrol. You can take up to three capsules by mouth three times a day for three weeks. PEA helps to stop physical and mental pain due to inflammation caused by cytokines in the body. PEA has the ability to decrease obsessive/compulsive (OCD) and suicidal thoughts within one to two days if taken at a high dose. Decreasing to a lower dose when your thoughts are stabilized, such as one capsule twice a day, is a good dose.

Waayb 10 mg/pump:

- For children **older than six years up to 12 years of age,** apply one pump to the base of the neck just below the hairline every night.

Waayb 5 mg/pump CBD (pure cannabidiols):

- For children **less than six years,** apply one pump to the base of the neck, just below the hairline, at bedtime, and rub in well.

Medline CBD 2000mg with Limonene, Active Daytime Recovery w/Limonene:

- For **teens or adults with autism** use this form of CBD using 0.5 to 1.0 ml every morning.

Tri-Fortify Watermelon or Orange Glutathione:

- Take one teaspoon a day.

Relax Max by Xymogen:

- Mix 1-2 scoops in water (to taste) and sip throughout the day.

H4H Adult Insomnia Kit:

OptiMag Neuro by Xymogen:

- 1-2 scoops mixed in water beginning around five pm.

Medline CBD with Myrcene (2000 mg):

- Take 0.5 to 1.0 ml about thirty minutes before bed if less than twelve years.

Neuro Night Essentials: follow the instructions on the bottle.

H4H Pediatric Insomnia Kit:

Melatonin Davinci Liposomal Spray:

- 1 to 2 squirts, not to be given after 3 a.m. One half-hour before bed, if they wake up another squirt can be given later on.

OptiMag Neuro by Xymogen:
- 1-2 scoops mixed in water beginning around five p.m.

H4H Adult Anxiety Kit:

Medline CBD with Limonene (2000 mg):
- Take 0.5 to 1.0 ml in the MORNING.

Relax Max by Xymogen:
- Mix 1-2 scoops in water (to taste) and sip throughout the day.

Triple Mag:
- 3 capsules two times per day.

H4H Pediatric Anxiety Kit:

Relax Max by Xymogen:
- Mix 1-2 scoops in water (to taste) and sip throughout the day.

H4H Pediatric Basics:

Dr. Paula's Fish Oil: 1 teaspoon daily.

Liquid Vitamin D3 with K2:
- Birth to four months, 1 drop every other day.
- Four months to one year, 1 drop a day.
- Beyond one year, 2 drops a day.
- Vitamin D levels will need to be run.

Activ Nutrients Chewable or Powder: (multivitamin) follow directions on the bottle.

H4H Adult Basics:

Vitamin D3 with K2 (5,000 IU): 1 capsule daily.

Activ Nutrients (multivitamin): follow instructions on the bottle.

Omaprem: 2 gel capsules per day.

H4H Adult Help-My-Gut Kit:

SBI Protect by Orthomolecular:
- Four capsules twice daily.
- Or 1 to 2 scoops two times per day.

OrthoSpore IgG by Orthomolecular:
- 3 capsules at bedtime.

SBI Protect by Orthomolecular: 1 scoop once to twice daily.

OrthoSpore IgG by Orthomolecular: 1 capsule at night.

The information is for informational purposes only, is not a substitute, and does not render medical or psychological advice, opinion, diagnosis, treatment, or cure. The information provided should not be used for diagnosing or treating a health problem or disease. It is not a substitute for professional care. Always seek the advice of your physician or other qualified healthcare providers with any questions you have regarding your medical conditions and treatment options.

Interpreting Your Genetic Code

Did you know that our genetic DNA code is 99 percent identical in all humans? SNPs (Single Nucleotide Polymorphisms) are actually what make you unique. In addition to traits like eye and hair color, SNPs affect other traits like B12 absorption, Vitamin A, D, and E conversion, caffeine metabolism, neurotransmitter production, bioavailability, and immune response, to name a few. It's important to note that SNPs are not good or bad; it's all about how these SNPs interplay with your nutrition and environment. In times of increased trauma, stress, poor nutrition or illness, these SNPs can turn on to overproduce or turn off and reduce function, placing people at risk of nutritional deficiencies, unable to detoxify from toxic substrates, have dysregulated metabolic hormones, or put a person at risk for an overactive immune response. Turning genes on or off is known as **Epigenetics.** Epigenetics is the study of how your behaviors and environment can cause changes that affect the way your genes work. When a SNP is being expressed and affecting function, knowing you can positively influence your genetic expression by modifying your environment and nutrition is empowering. Your environment is absolutely a predictor of health and well-being. That is why you start with modifying your environment (ERMI/Actino home testing), stress, nutrition, and lifestyle to create an inner and outer environment conducive to healing.

It's important to understand that SNPs are different from genetic mutations. Mutations create a predictable disease state like Cystic Fibrosis or Huntington's disease.

It is easy to feel unsure of how to pull together the many pieces that make up a comprehensive care plan. That is why Hope for Healing designed its healing journey to begin with lifestyle and next with nutrigenomics to deepen the personalization and steer clinical decision-making for the medical interventions. To learn more about Hope for Healing's Precision Genetics care path and order a cheek swab test kit, visit get2theroot.com and schedule a Welcome Call.

This intelligent sequential patient journey of lifestyle, genetics, and medical interventions is designed to help you receive the best return on investment.

"After nearly a decade of practicing functional medicine, we have designed this patient journey because we believe this is personalized medicine at its finest."
Paula Kruppstadt, MD

Part 2: The Stages of Change

Throughout the curriculum you will be identifying reasonable steps that are a match to your current ability (motivation + competence + confidence) and the changes that you have sufficient inspiration to change.

Dr. James Prochaska's book, *Changing to Thrive*, is a recommended reading. Dr. Prochaska teaches us there are five stages of change. You will be cycling through these stages of change throughout your functional medicine journey.

"Every success story is a tale of constant adaptation, revision, and change."
Richard Branson

It's Important to Know Action is Not the Only Step in Change.

It's equally as important to have *thinking* and *feeling* goals. Contemplating the pros and cons before deciding to layer in a modification is an important step in the change process. Taking time to prepare for a lifestyle or nutrition modification is also equally important to the action-oriented step in the change process. Actually, by honoring these two stages of change, action can feel more effortless and simpler. Now that's a formula for a sustained change!

1. **Pre-contemplation**: People can get stuck in pre-contemplation because they feel **doubtful,** they can change, they feel **demoralized** because they've tried before, or they **don't** know how to change. So, if there are habits you aren't ready to change, is it perhaps because of one of these three Ds? Being honest with yourself is essential in the healing process.

2. **Contemplation**: In this stage, a person recognizes the need to change behavior and intends to begin within the next six months. If you feel ambivalence or hesitancy regarding any lifestyle change, it is important to weigh the pros and cons. Pros: What is good about keeping things as they are now? Cons: What is bad about keeping things as they are now? Weigh the pros of not changing against the short and long-term pros of changing the behavior. Ideally, the pros of change win out. You will read more about Decision Balance in Chapter Three.

3. **Preparation**: What small things can you do to prepare for a larger change? What is just one thing you can do today?

4. **Action**: Remember motivation + competence + confidence equal action!

5. **Maintenance**: Once you make a change, maintain it so the other modifications can build upon your foundation. *Aka* stabilization!

In contrast, the secret to success is building momentum by making small changes that feel easy and within your current emotional and financial ability, sustaining those changes and repeating the process. These small changes add up to making big changes. Even if you *can* afford advanced medical interventions, this intelligent sequence helps prevent harm from ill-timed medical interventions plus optimizes the effectiveness of the treatments. There is ***no skipping*** the nutrition and lifestyle changes!

The definition of current ability is repeated throughout this workbook. Current ability means those changes you have sufficient motivation, confidence, and competence to successfully change. As you continue to work within your current ability and build upon success, you will eventually feel ready to layer in more advanced changes, like going 100 percent gluten-free.

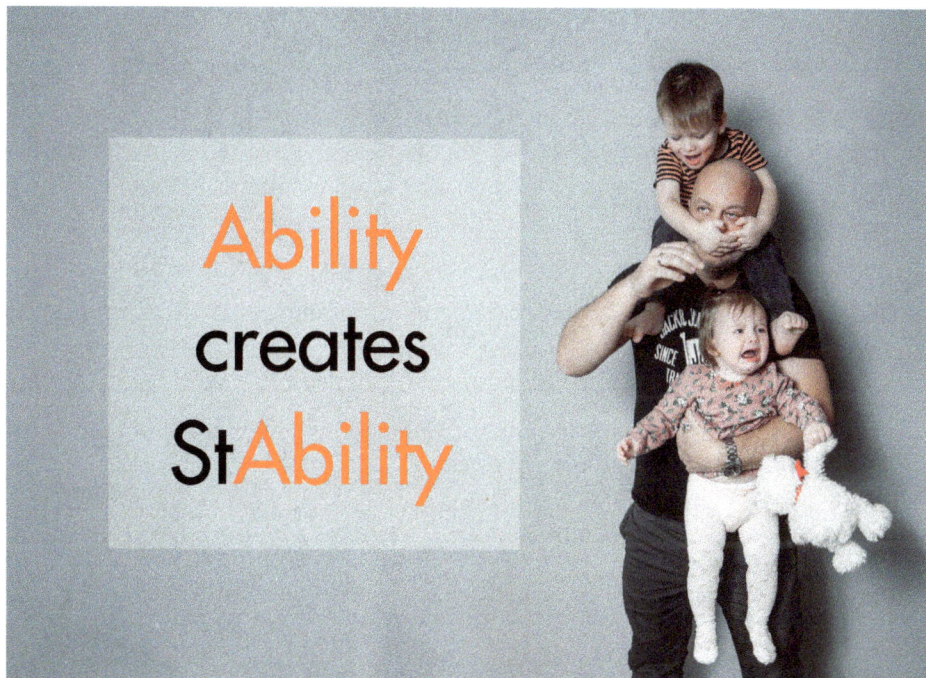

Some patients remove gluten for a month and say it didn't work. Others think a little bit of gluten won't hurt on occasion. And others will replace gluten with highly processed gluten-free packaged items. **This is referred to as the gluten-free crap trap!** If you are looking for immediate ROI by removing gluten, for example, then the point is being missed. <u>Gluten is just one source of inflammation</u>.

No one intervention alone will solve all pains. Removing x and expecting y to happen is not how it works. Remember, in the layering method, nutrition and lifestyle modifications, genetics, and medical protocols and therapies work in combination to reduce inflammation and restore your health and freedom. This layering method is what will provide the best results.

*It's to your advantage to already have gluten and dairy removed by the time you meet with your provider, but it doesn't need to be removed all at once. You can take a gradual approach. One method is to first work with ratios. For example, if your child is drinking milk, give them three-fourths cow's milk and one-fourth nondairy milk without carrageenan. Continue to adjust your ratios until the cow's milk has entirely been eliminated. Making lateral shifts is another recommended strategy. For example, instead of CheezIts© to Mary's Gone Cheezee Crackers©. It's okay if your child does not like the taste right away. Remain calm and understanding and ensure them that when they are ready you can try again. Your child is a picky eater, but removing the high- allergens will actually make them more accepting of nutrient-dense, healing foods.

As you create a solid foundation with the first two Rs, *removing* sources of inflammation and *replacing* them with clean, whole foods and natural products, then you will be ready to work with your provider and layer in the advanced medical interventions and functional therapies. This is how you use your time and money wisely and optimize your return on investment.

Functional Medicine is Personalized Because it's *Your* Plan!

Your life will happen—either accidentally or deliberately. You can hope that you'll accidentally fall into good health ... or you can deliberately make a plan and move toward your health goals and to experience well-being.

Use the Menu of Nutrition and Lifestyle Options at the back of the workbook to select changes that feel easy, so you can begin to gain momentum to eventually add in larger changes that perhaps feel challenging right now. As your confidence and commitment grow, what you once perceived as challenging *will* feel reasonable.

For any change, you're considering, rate it from one to ten based on how confident you feel about making the change. For any changes that you rate as less than seven, break it into smaller steps that you feel more confident and motivated to make! As mentioned earlier, eating 100 percent gluten- or dairy-free may not be your first step. The first step may be to first evaluate how much exposure you are currently having to these high-inflammatory foods. The next step may be to begin actively *reducing* your intake.

When you choose a change in your current ability, it feels good. When you feel good about what you are doing, you will naturally keep it as part of your care plan and look for more change you can do.

Chapter One Summary

Designing comprehensive and coordinated care plans that create consistency and continuity of care is a skill necessary to develop. A comprehensive plan may include but is not limited to mental, emotional, spiritual, nutritional, and lifestyle modifications, medical protocols, functional therapies, structural integration, vision, bodywork, and airway treatments. Select carefully what you can implement and sustain for the next ninety days. Ninety days give enough time to organize, implement, and stabilize the modifications and protocols before adding in the next round of modifications and protocols. Use the Menu of Nutrition and Lifestyle Options in the back of the workbook to choose those changes you have sufficient motivation and ability. Anchor the changes with a prompt, a habit you are already doing well, and remember to celebrate!

The secret to success is building momentum by making small changes that feel easy and within your current emotional and financial ability, sustaining those changes, and repeating the process. These small changes add up to make big changes. Even if you can afford advanced medical interventions, this intelligent sequence helps prevent harm from ill-timed medical interventions and optimizes the treatments' effectiveness. There is no skipping the nutrition and lifestyle changes. **Evolving ninety-day plans allow you to pace yourself. There is no rushing the body to heal from once thought dead-end diagnosis.**

If you have not yet purchased the Personalized Medicine Care Planner, visit Braughler Books. The care planner is your record-keeping journal, helping you track essential information about your functional medicine journey. Inside, you will find prompts to help you organize, document, track, and budget, as well as helpful advice on ways to partner with family, educators, and medical providers on your personalized ninety-day care plans.

Functional medicine is a journey, and any journey requires a map and a log to record your progress. Think of this workbook as your map and the care planner as your captain's log. The workbook guides your change process, and your care planner allows you to successfully track where you have been so that you can make informed decisions about the next steps.

Build Your Personalized Care Plan

What are you already doing well? What mindset, emotional, spiritual, nutritional, lifestyle, therapies, and medical interventions are you planning to layer in next? As you continue your journey, you will layer more changes to work in combination with the previous ninety-day plan.

Supplement, Rx, Medical Protocols

Therapies | Structural Integration | Bodywork

Modifiable Lifestyle Factors

Mental | Emotional | Spiritual

Chapter One Homework

Functional medicine is 80 percent nutrition and lifestyle and 20 percent well timed-medical interventions. Functional medicine's success is largely determined by how well a patient, or a parent can remove and replace sources of inflammation.

Journal about your intrinsic motivators. Intrinsic motivation involves doing something because it is both interesting and deeply satisfying. We perform such activities for the positive feelings they create, and they typically lead to optimal performances. Write your responses in the pages to follow. This is the starting point for Writing Your Story of Hope and Healing.

1. What does functional medicine mean to you?

2. Write down what you want to gain into your life from your functional medicine journey.

3. How do you want to feel in life?

4. What do you want to be surrounded by?

5. What does support look like to you?

6. How do you define success?

7. What is motivating you to be here, to pursue functional medicine?

8. What is your long-term goal?

9. Where would you like to be in three months, one year, five years?

10. What high-allergens are you eating each day?

11. How many times a week are you or your child eating fast food?

12. What lifestyle changes do you feel motivated to work on during the next three months? Be specific. (Reference the Menu of Nutrition and Lifestyle Options)

13. What do you need to implement your plan? Recipes, resources for specialized groceries, access to exercise equipment ...

14. Are these changes attainable in three months?

15. On a scale from one to ten, how realistic are the changes that you chose to implement in the next three months?

16. How will you measure your progress toward the accomplishment of nutrition and lifestyle changes?

17. What do you think about scheduling these changes Look ahead in your calendar for social outings or holidays that are coming up to begin to prepare. Later in the course, we discuss how to go against the cultural norm at holidays and parties and still enjoy them.

18. How do you want to be supported? What do you need to be successful?

Now, think about a time when you have started a new diet, fitness plan, and healthy lifestyle change.

1. Why did you start the plan?

2. What support was available to you?

3. What went well?

4. What challenges did you encounter?

5. What assisted you to overcome challenges?

Optional Homework

- Create a vision board if having a visual reminder helps stay connected to your intrinsic motivators. Most people create a vision board of things they want, and then quickly become upset that they are not immediately manifested. Rather than creating a vision of what you want, create a vision board of why you are changing, what is motivating you, what are you relying on, **and how you want to feel during this change process. This clarifies your vision for how you want to affect your circumstances.**

Chapter 2: Implementing Your Plan

Key Terms

Neuroplasticity: the brain can modify, change, and adapt its structure and function throughout life.

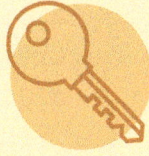

Self-Directed Neuroplasticity: is the mind's ability to change brain function through the power of thought.

Mind-Body Medicine: a health practice that combines mental focus, controlled breathing, and body movements to help relax the body and mind.

Fixed Mindset: the condition of people who believe their qualities and abilities are fixed and cannot change.

Growth Mindset: people believe they can develop their most basic abilities through dedication and hard work.

Brain-Heart Coherence: defined as a state in which the brain and heart work harmoniously to experience more emotional balance, sharper mental focus, increased resilience, and less stressful emotions.

Learning Outcomes

Part 1: Identity

- Evaluate your belief about your or your child's diagnosis.
- Compassionately observe your thoughts.
- Finding ingrained fixed mindsets.

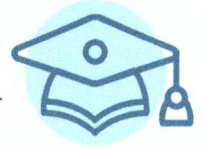

Part 2: Mental and Emotional Components of a Comprehensive Plan

- Utilizing neuroplasticity to create a mindset conducive to healing.
- Elevating your emotional state to affect your circumstances.
- Learning Mind-Body Medicine techniques.
- Acquiring skills to correct and stay the course during increased stress and chaos.

Part 3: Spiritual

- Acknowledging the spiritual role in healing.
- Finding sources of inspiration.

Introduction

Our brain is hardwired to scan for threats (which helped our ancestors survive), which means we are good at learning from bad experiences but relatively bad at learning from good ones. And because we humans have evolved to focus on potential threats to life or safety, we now tend to pay more attention to adverse situations, no matter how insignificant. Constant focus on negative experiences adversely affects emotional health and leads to "negative, limiting, and fear-based thought patterns," also known as deceptive brain messages. So, of course, you have self-sabotaging thoughts that fuel anxiety! This is normal!

Negative activities and structures in the brain usually do not just change for the better on their own; they are built into tissues whose structures tend to persist unless they are actively changed. Similarly, effectively positive activities and structures need to get built into the brain; they usually do not just develop on their own.

Dr. Rick Hanson: author and expert psychologist in the Neuroscience of Lasting Happiness teaches, we must level the playing field by using our minds to change our brains with deliberate effort. This is called self-directed neuroplasticity. We must train our minds to tune in and determine 'what am I thinking?' and is it serving my health and happiness? Or am I locked into my limbic brain, constantly scanning for threats of all kinds, and focused on survival?

This chapter focuses on the mental, emotional, and spiritual components of a comprehensive care plan to transform chaos, stress, and adversity. Positive Identities, Metacognition, Emotional Regulation, Emotional Intelligence, Neuroplasticity, Mind-Body Medicine, Breathing Exercises, Quantum Field Theory, and Brain-Heart Coherence will be discussed. The goal of this chapter is to reach for better-feeling thoughts deliberately and to nurture elevated emotions which positively influence your hormones, neurochemistry, genetic expression, the words you speak, behaviors, habits, character, and destiny.

Review

In Chapter One you began creating a three-month personalized nutrition and lifestyle plan based on your current ability (motivation + competence + confidence).

Remember, **overwhelm** is just a sign you are trying to do too much too fast. The layered approach of taking small steps incrementally that are decided upon based on your current ability and building on those small wins with the bigger goal in sight ensures success.

Choosing small incremental changes, that are a match to your current ability, and layered to work in combination, is the formula that prevents you from creating elaborate expectations for yourself that you can't reach. This is the antidote to feeling demoralized or doubtful you can positively affect your outcome. Take small deliberate steps, and over time, you will move closer and closer to your health goals.

Implementing Your Plan

Training your mindset and elevating your emotions to implement and sustain changes for the long journey of reversing chronic and degenerative conditions and becoming our best selves is where the rubber hits the road! Training the mind to create healthy habits and make informed decisions is as important to your plan as healing and strengthening the body.

> *"When it comes to your health, there is one factor that is more important than perhaps any other. If it is missing from your life, it causes or worsens 95 percent of all illness . . . It is the health of your mind and spirit."* Dr. Mark Hyman

Life **will** throw you curve balls while you are implementing your plan and you will want to revert back to familiar habits . . . this chapter's skills are how we will soften the effects of stress and other triggers that life throws at us so to remain committed to our family's care plan and journey.

We all usually have something very specific to be negative about in our life. Focusing on the symptoms makes you more and more miserable. When you think about your misery, talk about your misery, get other people to relate, and talk about their misery, the more specifically negative you are, the more resistance is created to prevent you from experiencing what you want. It is easy to get carried away with this.

Most people move into action without first aligning their breath, thoughts, and words with ideally what they would like to experience, with what they want to create! They are reacting to the chaos, therefore creating more chaos. This chapter teaches how to have the most power in our outcomes and neutralize the chaos!

Part 1: Identity

Common thoughts associated with chronic conditions or having a child diagnosed with autism or PANS/PANDAS is to feel guilt, shame, embarrassment, and anger. It's easy to feel like you are failing. With that in mind, let's redefine failure. Failure is a temporary setback, usually because we are *trying to do too much too soon*. Success is pursuing a worthwhile goal.

Many beliefs sabotage success because they keep a person in a fear/victim failure-like state. In this chapter, we work to acknowledge and transform limiting beliefs to move beyond feeling stuck.

Fear/victim mentality will only sabotage your healing effort and lock you in a mindset of lack and scarcity. Plus, fear is not a sustainable motivator.

Taking steps to shift away from feeling punished or forsaken, and learning to accept your diagnosis and/or past pains, allows you to be open to receiving the lessons to be learned from them. Being humble and learning what your current pains have come to teach is a necessary shift in your perspective. This shift in perspective is necessary so you can see your current symptoms/challenges as guides toward changing that which is no longer working for you. This is the path toward becoming your best self. I'm sure you have heard turn your "mess" into your "message." *Our greatest contribution often comes from our greatest pain*.

It can happen that a diagnosis becomes a person's identity. Your diagnosis **does not define** who you are. You are so much more than a collection of symptoms. This is where mindset and its connection with your health and well-being come into play.

The steps to create and support this shift can be bodywork like craniosacral work and lymphatic drainage, somatic emotional release, energy work, and coaching, all of which are other important components to a comprehensive care plan. Emotions get lodged in the body and we need help to bring those buried emotions to the surface to be released and ultimately transformed. It takes courage to bring the darkest parts of yourself out to the open. That's why having a collaborative care team is important to support you through this process and journey.

It's important to note that this also takes time and effort. It could be that things get worse before they get better as you move through this work. If you are prepared for this, then you can nurture yourselves through the healing process rather than thinking you are failing. Two steps forward, three steps back: it's like the ocean waves, or like a bow and arrow, you must pull back to flow forward.

A note for parents: you are also on a healing journey. Healing your past traumas, changing your nutrition and lifestyle, and transforming your mindset are equally as important as your child's health. This is a journey you are sharing with your child/children. Conventional and alternative interventions solely focus on the child. Until you embark on your own healing journey, your progress will be stifled.

Finding Fixed Mindsets

As mentioned, life will throw curve balls while you are implementing your plan. The curveballs are usually in the field of fixed mindsets *aka* limiting beliefs. Fixed mindsets can sound like this:

- I never get it right.
- This is so hard.
- How am I supposed to do all of this?
- My brain is hard-wired, this is just who I am.
- My child doesn't understand me.
- My child can't help himself.
- My child will not eat anything but his favorite foods.
- My child doesn't notice what I eat, so I can eat whatever I want.

Do any of these fixed mindsets resonate with you? When you are stressed, what repetitive and negative thoughts do you have? Compassionately observe your mind this next week. Observing your thoughts is called Metacognition. **Metacognition** is when you notice limited/limiting thoughts, objectify them by becoming the observer, and detach from them, unraveling yourself from the emotional threads that keep you locked in stress, fear, frustration, and overwhelm. Begin to document any limiting, fixed beliefs you hear yourself say, so you can work to transform them into thoughts that assist you in creating your health and freedom goals. You must decide what thoughts belong in your future.

"We see the world, not as it is, but as we are—or, as we are conditioned to see it." Stephen R. Covey

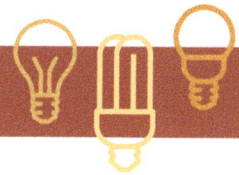

The Comprehension section is intended to optimize your comprehension. This section reviews the big ideas which make functional medicine provide the profound results we have come to expect. Think about what you have learned and how you will apply them to your unique and current circumstances.

Compassionately observe your mind this next week and document any limiting, fixed beliefs you hear yourself say.

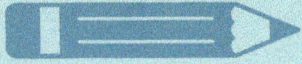

Being honest with yourself is the first step in genuine acceptance and a step closer to self-love. Just like your core, clinical imbalances provide invaluable clues to what you can do to regain balance, so do your thoughts.

What habits do you revert to when you are stressed?

What is the need behind the unhealthy coping strategy?

What is the feeling I am looking to gain from this coping strategy?

What thought and emotion is driving me to the need for the coping strategy?

Where is this thought coming from?

Did this thought come from someone else?

How can I take care of myself right now?

Neuroplasticity

Neuroplasticity is the ability of the brain to form and reorganize synaptic connections, especially in response to learning or experience or following injury. Neuroplasticity, also known as neural plasticity or brain plasticity, is the ability of neural networks in the brain to change through growth and reorganization.

Part of healing is neuroplasticity. The brain is AMAZING! It can modify, change, and adapt its structure and function throughout life. Toxicity and infections cause brain inflammation. When inflammation is removed, and essential vitamins and minerals are incorporated back into the body, the brain can change, leading to new neurons firing and wiring together, gaining function, and losing abnormal symptoms. This means that negative, limiting, fear-based self-deceptive messages can be reprogrammed with better-feeling thoughts that serve us in changing habits and creating our character and destiny. In this chapter, we talk about the Mental, Emotional, and Spiritual components of a comprehensive care plan that assist in rewiring, reprogramming, relearning, and reinventing a new self. Firing and wiring new circuitry in the brain to change your reality means you become greater than your circumstances.

> *"The rewiring, reprogramming is part of my story, too. I used to weigh almost 300 pounds and took antidepressants for ~twenty-seven years, but the principles of functional medicine combined with mind retraining has given me new life."*
> Paula Kruppstadt, MD

You cannot be ruminating about your problems and pain and expect to heal. The stronger the emotions you feel from some problem or condition, the more you can get pulled down into the underbelly of depression and fear. These thoughts are asking you to pay attention because where you place your attention is where you place your energy. And where you place your energy is what you create. **Emotional Intelligence** helps you stay present and create well-being throughout each day to change your thoughts, emotions, and environment, which modulates your gene expression. Oftentimes, it's past pain(s) and trauma(s) that interact with SNPs that tip you into your dis-ease state. Your dis-ease state affects your mindset and identity. This is why the timeline is so important and a valuable health analysis tool. You have to understand all the influencing factors in your life to reverse the physiological and emotional impact they have had on you. Therefore, nutrigenomics and some form of counseling and energy work are essential. Remember, health is primarily determined by the interplay of your stress, environment, nutrition, and genetic code.

Pay attention to the first thought you have in the morning. Train your mind to think thoughts of gratitude. Choose thoughts like, "What does greatness look like today? How would greatness act today?" Get excited! You can intentionally program your mind and that of your children's minds. What thoughts do you want to fire and wire together? How do you want to feel in life? **As Dr. Joe Dispenza says, *"You are installing new hardware, and when practiced enough, the hardware will become software and become the new voice in your head."*** And this voice is what programs the voice in your child's mind. Behaviors match intentions, therefore, your actions equal your thoughts. Construct thoughts you want to believe in and fire and wire those connections together. Self-regulate your emotions daily and change your emotional state on command to create balance and influence your circumstances.

A note to parents: You create your child's environment. Your stress, beliefs, thoughts, words, actions, and habits must be a part of their care plan to create an environment conducive to healing. This is a shared journey with your child, and you are leading by example. As you adopt this lifestyle and train your mind, you will become more matter of fact. **You will begin to parent your child rather than nurture your fear of the symptoms of their diagnosis.** Your children will feel this better emotional state and begin to synchronize with you. Your child will improve as you become more resilient, resourceful, and joyful. One of the best pieces of advice I received was that my children would mirror my habits.

"Become aware of the times you are fearful, nervous, deflated, frustrated, and anxious, and at that moment, decide to change your emotional state. To be independent of the conditions in your environment means you are mastering your environment, you are transforming fear into coherence and love, and wholeness, which is how you truly master your body and change your physiology." Dr. Joe Dispenza

---

Part 2: Mental and Emotional Components of Healing

Functional Mindset

Before you work on behavior change (Action), you must go upstream and deliberately direct your thoughts (Mind) and feelings (Emotional) and connect to your purpose and meaning (Spiritual).

Without prioritizing transforming your mindset, you will quickly resort to your ingrained perspectives and habits, which block your healing process.

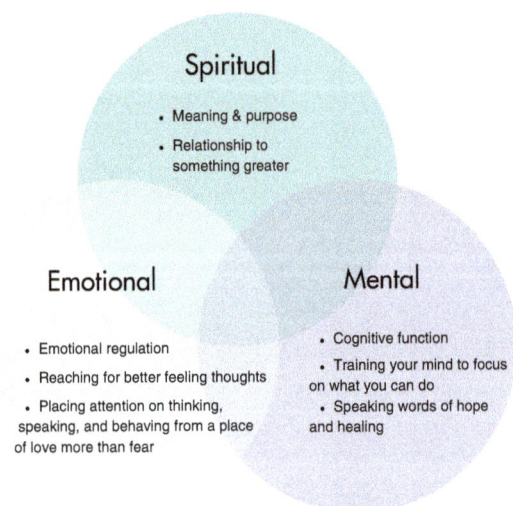

Spiritual
- Meaning & purpose
- Relationship to something greater

Emotional
- Emotional regulation
- Reaching for better feeling thoughts
- Placing attention on thinking, speaking, and behaving from a place of love more than fear

Mental
- Cognitive function
- Training your mind to focus on what you can do
- Speaking words of hope and healing

Let's recap quickly ...

Before we work on behavior change (action) we must go upstream and deliberately direct our thoughts and feelings ... If we try to change our behaviors without first changing our thoughts, feelings, and words, we will quickly resort right back to our ingrained habits.

Consciously paying attention to the thoughts running through your mind and the feeling they create is a priority. Notice what you are saying to yourself throughout the day.

Do you believe these thoughts? Are you shocked at how cruel the thoughts can be toward you? What do these thoughts remind you of? Did someone speak these words to you at one time? Are these thoughts serving you? Are you going to choose to continue tearing yourself down or choose better feeling thoughts?

Because of mental, emotional, and physical pain, we have all created coping strategies. Our coping strategies are telling us we need support. Your genetic code will provide great insight into what nutrients your body may have a higher demand for to help counterbalance the effects of stress and to better handle daily stressors and change. As you continue to remove sources of inflammation and train your mind, it will get easier to transform harmful behaviors to behaviors that are conducive to healing.

Mind-Body Medicine

Mind-Body Medicine uses the power of thoughts and emotions to influence physical health. You also have Mind-Body Medicine techniques to turn to as resources to help soften the effects of change and chaos associated with a complex diagnosis.

"The concept of total wellness recognizes that our every thought, word, and behavior affects our greater health and well-being. And we, in turn, are affected not only emotionally but also physically and spiritually." Greg Anderson

Mind-Body Medicine is how we transform coping strategies into self-care. A good question to ask yourself when you are reverting to old coping strategies is, *"How can I care for myself right now?"* Small little things, like breathing, making a cup of tea, going out into the shed, and screaming, are all ways to care for yourself and disrupt turning to old coping strategies.

We will explore breathing and other Mind-Body Medicine techniques coming up. The good news is there is so much you can do to support yourself in your change process.

Any repeated stimulus, whether positive or negative, has the potential to affect neuroplastic changes, ultimately leading to automatic responses or habits.

If you are noticing a habit, stop and ask yourself what is the thought, belief, or feeling that is driving me to this action? How are my words contributing to this habit? What do I need? What am I looking for? How can I take care of myself right now?

Being honest with ourselves is the first step in genuine acceptance and a step closer to self-love. After all, we can't hate ourselves and heal; we must train our minds to live in a state of acceptance and love.

"Negative thoughts and structures in the brain usually don't just change for the better on their own; they are built into tissues whose structures tend to persist unless they are actively changed. Similarly, effectively positive thoughts and structures need to get built into the brain; they usually don't just develop on their own." Rick Hanson, Ph.D.

Transforming Fixed Mindsets

Carol Dweck, PhD. developed the fixed versus growth mindset. A simple trick to transform fixed mindsets is adding the word *yet* to the end of your sentence. For example, I have not been able to be consistent with taking my supplements, *yet*. The yet leaves room for growth. You are working your way toward adopting and integrating that positive growth. Try it. It feels good!

Another researcher, Barbara Fredrickson, PhD is among the most highly cited scholars in Positive Psychology and is most known for her 1998 **"broaden-and-build theory of positive emotions."** Her theory is a blueprint for how pleasant emotional states, as fleeting as they are, contribute to resilience, well-being, and health. Dr. Fredrickson teaches that happiness is not something you have or don't have, but rather a skill that can be developed by broadening a repertoire of positive thought-actions, which allow individuals to see new possibilities, ideas, and opportunities thereby building and gaining new physical, social, and intellectual resources. The theory drives home the point that when you feel good about doing something then you are most likely to follow through with the action.

Gratitude is another tool to use to soften your resistance to change. Robert Emmons, the world's leading scientific expert on gratitude, says that "**Gratitude allows us to celebrate the present.** It magnifies positive emotions. Research on emotion shows that positive emotions wear off quickly. Our emotional systems like newness. They like a novelty. They like change. We adapt to positive life circumstances so that before too long, the new car, the new spouse, the new house—they do not feel so new and exciting anymore. But gratitude makes us appreciate the value of something, and when we appreciate the value of something, we extract more benefits from it; we are less likely to take it for granted. In effect, I think gratitude allows us to participate more in life. We notice the positives more, and that magnifies the pleasures we get from life. Instead of adapting to goodness, we celebrate goodness."

Functional medicine is a mutual-participatory medical model. Patients and parents are active participants in their journey to heal root causes and restore function. Dr. Emmon teaches that by practicing gratitude, you will become a greater participant in creating a mindset that grows and nurtures well-being.

To continue exploring the concept of neuroplasticity, and broadening and building happiness, we will dig deeper into self-directed neuroplasticity (SDN). This science teaches us about the mind's ability to change brain function through the power of thought and how thought can alter brain structure in overcoming habituated responses. This quote by Lao Tzu is a guide to help you move through your change process:

> *"Watch your thoughts, they become your words; watch your words, they become your actions; watch your actions, they become your habits; watch your habits, they become your character; watch your character, it becomes your destiny."*
> Lao Tzu

To follow Lao Tzu's guidance and change your thoughts/feelings to make a different action, you can use the Emotional Scale.

Love

Freedom | Appreciation

Joy | Knowledge | Empowerment |
Passion

Enthusiasm | Eagerness | Happiness

Positive Expectations | Belief

Optimisim

Hopefulness

Emotional Scale

Contentment

Pessimism

Train Your Mind.
Reach for better feeling thoughts.

Frustration | Impatience | Irritation

Overwhelm

Dissappointment

Worry

Anger

Blame

Revenge

Hatred | Rage

Jealousy

Insecurity | Guilt | Unworthiness

Fear | Grief | Depression | Despair | Powerlessness

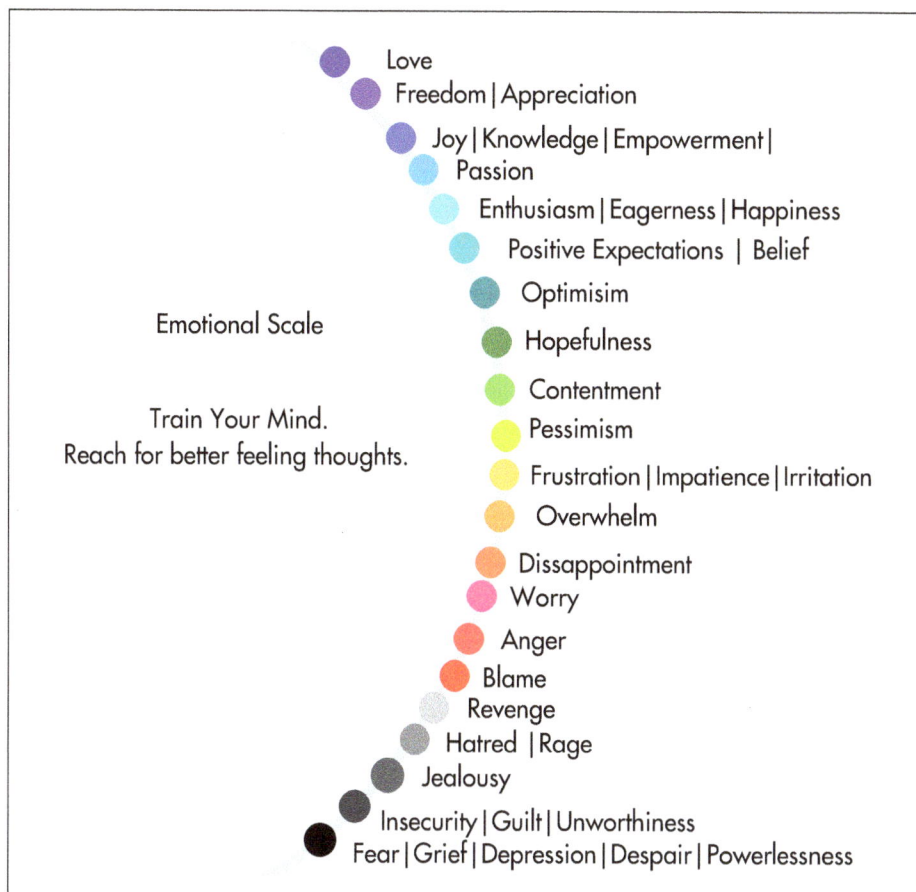

The Emotional Scale: An exercise to train your thoughts, and feelings to positively affect your words, actions, and habits.

Most of us are in a state of fear. The world is often a scary place. Illness keeps us locked in a fearful state. It's scary when our bodies and minds are out of balance. It is terrifying when our children are in pain.

We now know humans have evolved to focus on potential threats to life or safety. This means we are hard-wired to pay more attention to negative/adverse situations, no matter how insignificant. This constant focus on negative/adverse experiences adversely affects emotional health and leads to "negative, limiting, and fear-based thought patterns" also known as deceptive brain messages.

Moving from fear to love is a process. You cannot get to love from fear in one step. You must incrementally work your mind up the emotional scale. This scale helps to train your mind to have a perspective that's conducive to healing. Lao Tzu teaches us before we can change our actions and habits, we need to first change our thoughts.

To have self-care behaviors we need to have self-care thoughts. This means we need to change our perspective actively, and deliberately.

Here is a definition of love that may be helpful: love is curiosity, acceptance for what it is, and compassion. Another definition that was helpful to me is joy: feeling grateful even when things are not going my way.

I've often seen patients doing all the "right" things, yet they are angry and resentful, and therefore, they don't ever feel like they are making progress.

In the absence of a positive focus, a negative climate will become the norm: a constant state of anger, jealousy, and fear. These thoughts and feelings will keep appearing. You have a choice whether you allow these lower feelings to be imprinted and infuse your atmosphere and identity and influence the words you speak to your loved ones.

The Emotional Scale gives you a clear path on how to reach for better feeling thoughts, to choose more healing actions, and create habits that ultimately create your healing destiny. The nutrition and lifestyle changes you have chosen must be done mindfully, lovingly, with the intention that with each thought and each action you are creating an atmosphere of well-being.

"If you want to heal your heart's wounds, start healing your thoughts."
Alexandra Vasiliu

You can't jump from anger to optimism. You must work your way up the scale incrementally to train your mind to reach for a better feeling thought. This is to be practiced, throughout your day. If an emotion doesn't resonate with you, skip over it. After a while, you will be able to do this quickly in your mind.

A solution is not found by thinking and perseverating on the problem. This exercise guides you to find new ideas, thoughts, inspirations, and solutions to shape and steer your healing journey. This exercise helps you to lean into love, the greatest reason and motivator. It is a method to airlift you out of fear and allow love to be the underpinning to your decisions, actions, habits, character, and destiny.

This is how you begin to affect your environment rather than reacting to the chaos and fear.

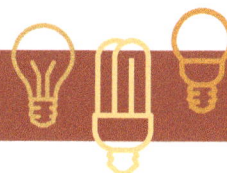

The Comprehension section is intended to optimize your comprehension. This section reviews the big ideas, which make functional medicine provide the profound results we have come to expect. Think about what you have learned and how you will apply it to your circumstances. Become conscious of what you are thinking and feeling and reprogram, reconstruct, and rewire new synaptic connections to think of new ideas, see new options, and create new results.

Write down common thoughts you hear yourself say using the emotions on the scale. For example, *"I'm jealous that my friends' toddlers are talking and able to participate joyfully in Mommy and Me outings."* **or** *"I'm stupid. I never get anything right."*

Next, work your way incrementally up the emotional scale. From jealousy, reach for rage, anger, or worry and write those thoughts down. Keep going as far as you can up the scale, practicing choosing your words to communicate authentically from this elevated emotional state.

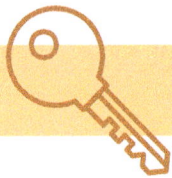

The more you practice reaching for better feeling thoughts you will begin to see your philosophy of healing emerging. Your better feeling thoughts become positive-guiding thoughts and affirmations. We refer to these positive affirmations as **key concepts.**

From your emotional scale exercise, create your key concepts: *your* philosophy to healing. Turn to your key concepts to catch yourself when you begin to a downward spiral into negative emotions.

Relying on your key concepts to interrupt and help you shift your emotional state is how you create the internal and external healing atmosphere! What consumes your thoughts controls your life.

Write Your Key Concepts

Pair the Emotional Scale Exercise with a Breathing Exercise

Stress fosters shallow breathing which makes thinking and decision-making feel more challenging than it needs to be. Notice your beathing throughout the day. Do you tend to hold your breath? In addition to training our minds, you also need to train your breathing patterns. This is one reason why yoga is an important healing modality.

Pair the emotional scale exercise with a breathing technique to integrate that better feeling thought into your inner voice! By inserting short pauses during the breath, moments of stillness in the body can create stillness in the mind. These moments of stillness help to create distance from a thought, emotion, or habit that is no longer of service or is fear based.

Segmented Breathing Exercise

- Arrange the body in a comfortable seated position with the spine tall, eyes soft or closed and allow the body to relax. Your back should be supported, and your feet should comfortably touch the ground.

- Bring your awareness to your natural breath for five to ten full breath cycles. Notice the quality of the natural breath. Are there pauses or catches in the inhale, in the exhale?

- Bring balance to the inhale and exhale where they are equal in length and quality. Do this without straining or effort. If one breath feels too long then shorten both breaths. You may be inhaling for a count of four, exhaling for a count of four, or inhaling six, exhaling six. Continue for a few rounds of breath.

- Once your balanced breathing is established, introduce the pauses. Inhale 50 percent, pause the breath, inhale another 50 percent, pause the breath, exhale 50 percent, pause the breath, exhale 50 percent, pause the breath.

Segmented Breathing Exercise with Counts

Four count breaths

Inhale for two counts (50 percent), pause the breath for two counts, inhale for two counts (50 percent), pause the breath for two counts, exhale for two counts (50 percent), pause the breath for two counts, exhale for two counts (50 percent), pause the breath for two counts.

Six count breaths

Inhale for three counts (50 percent), pause the breath for three counts, inhale for three counts (50 percent), pause the breath for three counts, exhale for three counts (50 percent), pause the breath for three counts, exhale for three counts (50 percent), pause the breath for three counts.

Continue breathing with pauses for ten full rounds.

Allow the breath to return to its natural rhythm and pay attention to any sensations, thoughts and emotions that may be present.

You may want to journal after this practice.

Simply bringing awareness to your breath is accessible at any time during your day and is one of the quickest ways to focus, calm, and become present.

Breathing Prayer and 4-7-8 Breathing

Dr. Andrew Weil originated the 4-7-8 Breathing Technique.

If you are sitting upright, make sure that your feet are comfortably placed flat on the ground and that your back is supported. You may also lie flat on your back to do this exercise. Relax and become conscious of your breath. Breathe in through your nose for about the count of four (a more rapid inhale), hold your breath for a count of seven, then breathe out for the count of eight through your lips. As you breathe out, purse your lips as if you were breathing out through a straw. Do this several times, paying close attention to the inhale, the holding of air, then deliberately blowing out for twice as long as your inhalation breath. Doing this cycle of 4-7-8 breathing for five to seven times tends to move you rapidly from a sympathetic to parasympathetic (rest and digest) status.

Once you've relaxed, do the following with the 4-7-8 breaths.

This breathing prayer exercise is from *The Ruthless Elimination of Hurry*, a book by John Mark Comer.

Breathe out Anger and breathe in Love.

Breathe out Sadness and breathe in Joy.

Breathe out Anxiety and breathe in Peace.

Breathe out Fear and breathe in Trust.

Breathe out The Need to Control and breathe in Detachment (an inner measurement that God is guiding and I am not).

Breathe out Discontentment and breathe in Contentment.

This 4-7-8 breathing exercise and breathing prayer should take no more than about five to seven minutes total.

4-7-8 breathing is excellent for going to sleep at night, lying in your bed!

Practical Application

The emotional scale and segmented breathing exercises are to be quickly done several times a day throughout the day. This is how you train your mind, emotions, and breathing to lead you out of the dark hole of despair that illness brings. Remember, your actions will follow. **So before trying to change your habits, *first train your mind, emotions and your breath*.**

It may only feel like anger, but if you've come from depression then anger can feel sweet. Anger is more toward joy on the emotional scale than fear. Some people think it is worse to feel angry, but with the right support, anger is a step we need to move through on our way to joy.

It's ok to feel the fear based deceptive thoughts. Remember, it's normal! It's ok to be angry. We just don't want to get stuck there. Having a safe place to express our anger, where we can 'lose our mind' is an important part of healing. The key phrase is 'having a safe place'. Misplaced anger destroys relationships and the kind of anger that comes with a chronic disease does and will be expressed. Make it a priority to find safe places to release pent-up anger so the emotional scale exercise feels more authentic.

We must love ourselves before we can genuinely heal. To love ourselves, we must accept that we are exactly where we are supposed to be, doing exactly what we are supposed to be doing. We must make every thought, every word, and each movement deliberate and grounded in love. This chapter's lessons teach how to apply the lifestyle and nutrition changes into your unique and current circumstances. Knowing how to apply information is knowledge and knowledge is empowering. The goal is to find love and joy even during agony and defeat. Both love and joy are not determined by our circumstances. Love is who we are; we are just covered up with our symptoms of dis-ease. You are learning how to uncover yourself!

Place more emphasis on loving yourself, coaching yourself through this process rather than focusing on the fear that ensues from chronic disease. Place priority on who you are becoming rather than your end, desired goals.

Healing is a decision to see love where we saw fear before. It's a shift in perception and a choice to be compassionate. It is common to focus so much on wanting that end goal of relief and recovery from our symptoms/diagnosis. Wanting something other than what we have at this exact moment is a real source of anxiety and depression. Working on loving what you are doing right now and trusting that all these small steps, done in love, will accumulate to make big changes is a method worth considering. A lot of positive change can happen in one year!

> *"To be content doesn't mean you don't desire more, it means you're thankful for what you have and patient for what's to come."* Tony Gaskins

Remember what makes functional medicine unique is the mental/emotional/spiritual components in addition to the physical lifestyle changes. As you remove sources of inflammation, this work becomes much, much easier! Your thinking becomes clear. You can find joy more easily even if life isn't currently what you had wanted it to be.

These exercises also can set you up for meditation. Feel your breath, feel the emotions from your better feeling thoughts in your body. Appreciate your willingness and devotion to training your mind. Practicing this throughout the day directs your words. And your actions follow your thoughts and your words. This is actively creating neuroplasticity.

PARTS Work by Internal Family Systems, Dick Schwartz

PARTS Work: we often speak about our emotions from the place of "I." I am angry, I am hurt, I am in pain, I am sick ... By reframing the statements from I to "a part of me" you can move toward creating self-space and be less identified with the emotion ... For example

> I am frustrated because of my flare-up *versus* a part of me feels frustrated because of my flare-up.

Use the emotional scale to move toward a better feeling thought

- Curiosity – why does that part feel frustrated? What belief, emotion, or sensation is there right now?
- Acceptance – ahh, okay, this has come to teach me something, what can I learn? What is one thing I can do to positively affect my circumstance? ...
- Compassion – don't be so hard on myself! No judging.

Part 3: Spiritual

Spirituality is many things to different people.

Spirituality: the sense of connectedness with "something higher"—an absolute, immanent, or transcendent power. Spirituality also is about meaning and purpose. In a National Library of Medicine article, The Meaning of Healing: Transcending Suffering, the author Thomas Egnew writes "Healing was associated with themes of wholeness, narrative, and spirituality. Healing is an intensely personal, subjective experience involving a reconciliation of the meaning an individual ascribes to distressing events with his or her perception of wholeness as a person."

"Spirituality is recognizing and celebrating that we are all inextricably connected to each other by a power greater than all of us, and that our connection to that power and to one another is grounded in love and compassion. Practicing spirituality brings a sense of perspective, meaning, and purpose to our lives." Brene Brown

Quantum Physics

Quantum Physics is a branch of physics that connects science, psychology, and spirituality and demonstrates that the world and our role in it are malleable to human choice and awareness. Dr. Joe Dispenza is a researcher, lecturer, author, and corporate advisor who teaches how to harness the power of quantum physics. Quantum physics makes the point that energy and matter are one and the same; because they are the same, your mind (energy) can change the body (matter).

Dr. Joe's key message is that when you continuously think the same thoughts, which conjure the same emotions, you nurture the same neurochemistry, which produces the same hormones, signaling the same genetic expression which ultimately creates the same choices, the same actions/behaviors, and you experience the same results. He says this way of thinking, feeling, and behaving becomes so familiar you don't even know it can be different.

"The definition of insanity is doing the same thing and expecting different results." Albert Einstein

Habits are frequent repetitive thoughts running on autopilot, locking you into a reactive state that keeps life the same, leaving people feeling victimized and helpless by their circumstances. Dr. Joe says, *"Most people love to tell the story of their past. I am asking you to tell the story of your future. When the brain is no longer a record of the past, it becomes the map of the future. The process of transformation and change is going from one state of body/mind to another."* This means you must revisit your beliefs and question whether they serve or hinder you.

Dr. Joe has numerous books like *Breaking the Habit of Being Yourself* and *Becoming Supernatural* and online courses like The Formula©.

"Light a match in a dark place, become conscious of what you think and feel, and learn how to reprogram your mind to see new options and think new ideas." Dr. Joe Dispenza

---

Instead of waiting to feel joy, satisfaction, happiness, success, and abundance, you must look for more ways to feel these feelings now and imprint the feelings into every action and interaction to cause an effect. Most people are waiting for something outside themselves to help them feel good. A great site to visit to learn more about the research behind cultivating emotional intelligence to affect your hormones, neuro-chemistry, genetic expression, and personal reality is https://drjoedispenza.com/pages/scientific-research.

"So much of what we talked about in yesterday's coaching session spoke to me. I need to focus on her and not her diagnosis. I must parent and love her and not make it all about the autism. Talk to her like she understands. Let her see me laugh and enjoy life, and that finding happiness and joy leads to recovery.

"I feel like I've been on a mission since my son was born and since my daughter came home with us to give them every chance to improve and succeed, and I've lost sight of what's important. Thank you so much!" Michelle M., parent

---

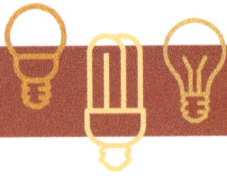

The Comprehension section is intended to optimize your comprehension. This section reviews the big ideas which make functional medicine provide the profound results we have come to expect. Think about what you have learned and how you will apply them to your unique and current circumstances.

Define self-directed neuroplasticity.

What Mind-Body Medicine techniques are you already using? What new ones did you learn?

What does the spiritual role in healing mean to you?

Describe how you imagine using these skills to stay the course in times of increased stress and chaos.

Correcting and Staying the Course

At first, you are excited. Yes! I'm going to do this! Then, life slaps you in the face. Life becomes way more chaotic. This feels like the worst time to begin this care plan. You may run into every single doubter you know. People may even say you are crazy. Well-intended family members can sabotage your efforts. You may even hear it is unsafe to eliminate entire food groups. You may hear what you are doing is just another fad diet. Your or your child's symptoms could be feeling like they are getting worse! Your cravings are raising their ugly, dominant head. You may very well find yourself wanting to revert to familiar habits ... this is all actually really normal.

In this chapter, you learned important skills to soften the effects of stress and other life triggers and transform the chaos to correct and stay on course with implementing your plan. Breathe! Rome was not built in a day. Restoring your or your child's body and mind to work correctly will take TIME. Remember that this is a marathon, not a sprint. If you are seeing your symptoms become worse, you are more than likely doing your homework. When we begin to address the underlying medical conditions, we usually can feel worse than better at first. When you ask your body to work differently than what you have grown accustomed to, it can become uncomfortable. Change is uncomfortable. This is why layering these interventions in an intelligence sequence, which is included in this workbook, is so important. They all must work in combination to restore clinical imbalances and heal psychological and physiological harm.

What do you do when you experience a setback? Quit? Is that what you would teach your children? No! Learn more, persevere, and grow through it! Reverting back to old habits is common as you build consistency and conviction to live your personalized care plan. Think of ways to reset yourself, like dancing, walking outside barefoot, watching funny movies as a family, and meditating. Conviction is a feeling of being certain about something. Conviction shows us the problem, separates us from it, and shows us the way out. One of a leader's greatest attributes is the ability to lead with conviction. Leaders with a strong sense of who they are and what they believe in and who allow those values and principles to come through in how they think, feel, and behave **will** correct and stay their course.

> **Regressions:** When you ask the body to perform differently, albeit better, it can trigger a regression. Keep going! Support yourself with Epsom salt baths, dry brushing, drinking bone broth and herbal teas and hydrating, breathing exercises, saunas, funny movies, gentle movement, soft lighting, etc. Check your care planner to see what supplement you added last and reduce the frequency you are giving it. Find ways to be gentle and encouraging to yourself as you walk this path of transformation.

"Many of life's failures are people who did not realize how close they were to success when they gave up." Thomas Edison

Chapter Two Summary

Albert Einstein is famous for saying, *"Information is not knowledge."* The gap between information and knowledge is to know how to apply the information confidently and competently to your unique circumstances to create positive change deliberately.

As you improve your Emotional Intelligence with metacognition, positive identities, self-directed neuroplasticity, quantum physics, and breathing exercises, next, practice creating brain-heart coherence. **Brain-Heart Coherence** is a state in which the heart, mind, and emotions are synchronized and balanced. This state is associated with feelings of well-being, relaxation, delight, satisfaction, and improved cognitive function. The term coherence implies harmonious order, connectedness, stability, and efficient use of energy that brings out the best in us.

Release being focused on your outcome and instead practice being present in a state of tranquility, support, satisfaction, enjoyment, delightedness, and surprise that is bigger than your immediate scenarios. **Training your mind and your nervous system to know what love feels like, to observe life through the lens of the heart, to reach for better-feeling thoughts and elevated emotions, and imprint your words and actions with love is what truly allows you to enjoy the present moment, even when it looks different than what you want.** This is how you stop doing what everyone else is doing and tap into your intuition, your higher knowing of what is right for you and your family!

This is ultimately the purpose of meditating, to lean back into a supportive, comforting, trusting energy where you can access the feeling of unconditional love. Dr. Joe Dispenza says, *"It's commonly accepted that when we are connected to the heart's inner knowing, its wisdom can be used as a source for love and higher, intelligent guidance. **The problem is that often the elevated feelings of the heart occur through chance— dependent upon something external in our environment—rather than something we can produce on demand.***

Instead of letting fear, impatience, or resentment grab hold of you to the point you feel nervous and think you have no control, practice opening your focus to the space around you, calibrate to a greater threshold of coherence, master the next moments, and ultimately you will master yourself. This is how you create an atmosphere around you that is conducive to healing. Our chronic conditions and our children demand us to learn mindfulness, which means being in the present moment. Depression tends to be about thoughts of the past, and anxiety tends to be induced by thoughts of the future. When you practice rooting the present moment in a state of love while you continue to balance nutritional, neurological, and biological imbalances, your and your child's anxiety and resistance **will** lessen. It is in this state you will find the **immediate** strengths and resources available you need each moment. As Ram Dass says, *"Be Here Now."* You are creating your future with this present moment. Choose to be love and watch your external circumstances shift.

HeartMath Institute researchers have shown that positive emotions—such as gratitude, joy, and compassion—can lead to beneficial changes in gene expression that affect our immune function, inflammation, and more.

"I realized my children were growing up without hearing their mom laugh. I decided to bring laughter back into our home. The first time I practiced laughing, my youngest son began crying. I must have sounded pretty delirious. The more I practiced returning laughter and joy into our day-to-day moments, and the more I infused love into every small action, from washing the dishes to brushing my teeth to putting my children's shoes on, I noticed everyone started to get better. I trusted that if I could train myself to live in a state of love, while living our transformational journey, all of these small, seemingly inconsequential daily activities would accumulate over time to make a big change. And they did! In learning to love what was before me even when it was terrifying, I did what many still say is impossible." Kara Ware

Build Your Personalized Care Plan

What are you already doing well? What mindset, emotional, spiritual, nutritional, lifestyle, therapies, and medical interventions will you layer in next? As you continue your journey, you will layer more changes to work in combination with the previous ninety-day plan.

Supplement, Rx, Medical Protocols

Therapies | Structural Integration | Bodywork

Modifiable Lifestyle Factors

Mental | Emotional | Spiritual

Chapter Two Homework

We take for granted and, in the most part, are not even aware of the 60,000 plus thoughts per day fired by electrical impulses through our brain. We rarely question what is generating these electrical charges, igniting our billions of neuronal connections. Surely, we are due to ask these questions. The following exercises should take no longer than ten minutes. You have time for this.

Journal prompt:

First, use your breathing exercise

1. Self-Directed Neuroplasticity exercise: use the emotional scale and work to find better feeling thoughts. Write down your key concepts: your philosophy of healing. Construct the thoughts you want to believe in, that you want to fire and wire.

More Homework Suggestions:

2. PARTS homework: a part of me is ... then use the breathing techniques and breathe into these parts of you. Invite love to come into the part of you that feels locked down. As you breathe, find your better feeling thought to help this part of you heal.

3. Gut check your plan and adapt. Make sure your plan is reasonable. Make a list of what you are doing that's working and what feels hard.

   a. Either break down the nutrition and lifestyle change that feels harder into smaller steps or perhaps even move the nutrition or lifestyle change to future considerations. You will get there, by taking these small steps and building on success.

      i. Place what feels hard in the next three months ... you can go back to it. As your competence and confidence grow, you will naturally be able to do what at one time felt impossible.

4. What does your future life look like, feel like? What does greatness look like, feel like?

Chapter 3: Sustaining Your Plan

Key Terms

Decision-Balance: "balance sheet" of comparative potential gains and losses.

Nonviolent Communication (NVC): is an approach to communication-based on principles of nonviolence.

CIRS Biomarkers: the lab markers evaluate how your environment may be affecting your health and causing symptoms.

Tick-Borne Complete: assesses for tick-borne diseases such as Lyme, Bartonellosis, Babesiosis, and Anaplasmosis.

Neural Zoomer: assesses circulating autoantibodies in the bloodstream that attacks the brain, nerves, and blood-brain barrier. This helps to evaluate PANS/PANDAS.

GI Map: evaluates for a multitude of bacterial, fungal, viral, and parasitic pathogens within someone's gut. It also evaluates the normal bacterial flora, enzyme balance, and overall gut health.

OAT Test: the purpose of the Organic Acid Test is to evaluate a person's metabolic health. It evaluates vitamin and mineral levels, oxidative stress, and neurotransmitter levels.

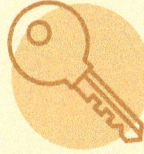

Learning Outcomes

Part 1: Functional Medicine is Another Word for Investment

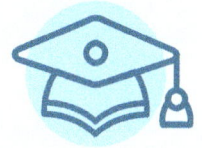

- Introducing the new modifiable lifestyle factors: time and money!
- Budgeting your time and money.
- Shifting your mindset regarding time and money.
- Optimizing your Return on Investment (ROI).
- Finding Financial Freedom.
- Using the Decision-Balance exercise to weigh the pros and cons of investing.
- Finding your voice to co-create your reasonable, personalized care plan.
- Planning time to stabilize changes.

Part 2: Communication and Interpersonal Skills to Build Better Relationships

- Communicating with your inner circle regarding changes: How do you go "against the norm" without alienating your family, inner circle, and work colleagues?
- Embracing Nonviolent Communication skills.
- Relying on Character Strengths.
- Communicating with integrity with the Hope for Healing Collaborative Care Team.
- Preparing to Tell Your Story!

Introduction

This chapter we focus on acquiring skills to sustain your personalized, comprehensive care plan. The new modifiable lifestyle factors, time, and money are introduced. To sustain your functional medicine journey, you will prioritize and plan to direct your time and money. We will explore communication and interpersonal skills to assist you in going against the cultural norm to build better relationships. This chapter wraps up with planning to tell your story and preparing to be an effective partner with your medical provider.

Review

You made your three-month modifiable nutrition and lifestyle change plan, gut-checked your plan and tweaked it to meet your current ability, and then you started training your mind and breathing to help with successful implementation. Plus, you have identified strengths, Mind-Body Medicine techniques, sources of inspiration, and support systems that can help when life throws you curve balls!

We all know what we need to do, however, implementing the changes when we don't feel well, and when our world is turned upside down is the crux. Before we work on behavior change (action) we must go upstream and deliberately direct our thoughts and feelings ... If we try to change our behaviors without first changing our thoughts, feelings, and words, we will quickly resort right back to our ingrained habits.

Most of us are in a state of fear. The world is often a scary place. Illness keeps us locked in a fearful state. It's scary when our bodies and minds are out of balance. It is terrifying when our children are in pain. And since we are hard-wired to pay more attention to negative/adverse situations and can easily get stuck in 'negative, limiting fear-based thought patterns', we can better understand the importance of training our minds to reach for better feeling thoughts. The techniques you learned in Chapter 2 are how you stop reacting to the chaos and instead positively influence your current circumstances.

Moving from fear to love is a process. You cannot get to love from fear in one step. You must incrementally work your mind up the emotional scale. This scale helps to train your mind to have a perspective and create an atmosphere that's conducive to healing. To have self-care behaviors we need to have self-care thoughts. This means we need to change our perspective, thoughts, and words actively, and deliberately.

A solution is not found by thinking and perseverating on the negative/adverse problem. If you are noticing a habit, stop and ask yourself what is the thought or feeling that is driving me to this action? How are my words contributing to this habit? What do I need? What am I looking for? How can I take care of myself right now? This is the formula for changing behaviors and habits.

You have now acquired skills to airlift you out of fear and allow love to be the underpinning of your decisions, actions, habits, character, and destiny. This is how you have the most power in your desired outcome!

An important reminder: Stabilization is the most overlooked facet of a comprehensive care plan. It is highly recommended that you plan for time to stabilize your changes, integrate them fully into your lives, fully complete protocols, prior to evolving your personalized care plan.

Part 1: Functional Medicine is Another Word for Investment

When working with a financial investor, it's highly likely you have heard them say,

"Successful investors act continuously on a plan rather than reacting to current events."

or

"By acting continuously on a rational plan, rather than reacting to current events, we have the best chance for long-term investment success."

At the beginning of your workbook, we introduced the concept that functional medicine is a new investment portfolio. We have accepted the social custom to invest in investment portfolios. How are you making a long-term investment plan for your functional medicine journey?

Since the process (journey) of removing the sources of inflammation, repairing physiological harm, and healing emotional traumas takes *time*, we must think of functional medicine as a long-term investment portfolio. Here's another thing you may have heard a financial investor say:

"Wise investors are committed to long-term gains rather than short-term wins!"

It's highly likely you are here because the path of insurance-covered services is not working and since insurance does not accept functional medicine, it can quickly become expensive!

The expense can be a big concern. But have you really done the math?

What is the financial impact of not changing? What lies ahead? If you did not follow the functional medicine path, what would the future look like?

Surgeries? A lifetime of prescriptive medicines? Not being productive at work or loss of employment? Recurring ER/urgent care visits and hospitalizations? Not being able to care for your adult autistic child? Think about how much you have spent in the past on your health or illnesses. Do you have medical debt? What has the chronic condition cost you beyond medical bills? Finances and budgets can cause friction in life: marriages suffer, and relationships suffer.

New Modifiable Lifestyle Factors: Time and Money

Along with the obvious lifestyle factors of nutrition, movement, relationships, sleep, and stress reduction, **time and money** must be considered. *Schedules and finances are sources of inflammation.* Reducing stress, worry, and uncertainty around time and money needs to be an important consideration when creating your care plan.

Schedules and budgets are synonymous with having a plan. Making a meal plan that puts too much pressure on your wallet and schedule is not setting yourself up for success.

Signing up for an expensive gym membership may work as a motivator in the beginning, but if it doesn't fit into your schedule or budget, it will become a source of guilt, shame, and embarrassment.

Stop and gut-check your plan again. Is it compatible with your time and financial thresholds?

How well do you triage your family's calendar? Is your schedule reasonable or are you doing way too much, spreading yourself thin, and adding to your inflammatory load? Busyness can be a disease in and of itself.

Parents can feel like they are failing because their kids are not in many activities or therapies ... is this true? There's that shame and guilt again! Children can be in so many therapies, that the parents are spending more time *'ubering'* than at home cooking and nourishing their families.

Functional medicine is larger than doctor's visits, supplements, labs, and testing; to sustain this way of living, you must be sure to work within your current financial threshold and reevaluate busy schedules.

Your relationship with time and money are sensitive topics yet must be included in a comprehensive care plan. These are important topics to consider exploring in more one-to-one health coaching sessions!

Budgeting Time and Financial Priorities

If you truly want to place your symptoms into remission and live the life you imagined, then start with deliberately casting your vote by directing your time and money toward living a lifestyle that will allow functional medicine to be successful.

Before getting started with the action of creating your time and money budget, let's first work on your mindset.

Take a moment to evaluate your beliefs around your functional medicine investment. Are you hearing yourself say any of these fixed mindset thoughts or fear-based emotions of lack and scarcity?

1. Eating healthy is expensive.
2. I can't afford that.
3. It is too expensive.
4. My child is in so many therapies I don't have time to cook.
5. I live alone. Cooking for one exacerbates my loneliness and seems wasteful.

Budget is another word for plan. Many patients jump into functional medicine and then quickly decide they cannot *sustain* the time it takes to prepare meals, include movement into their daily routine, and afford out-of-pocket diagnostic labs, supplements, and provider visits.

I have worked with clients that realized they were spending $300 on wine clubs each month. One family was spending $700 on fast food each month to sustain their child's autism therapy schedule (ABA, PT, OT, and speech therapies). Once these funds were redirected towards their functional medicine plan, and time was spent preparing meals, they found they were able to sustain their care and nurture their healing lifestyle.

Schedules are stressful—stress breeds dis-ease. Yikes! Where is your time going? Consider where you are spending your time; time is currency!

Look at the last couple of weeks on your calendar and create time categories. What categories fill most of your time? Children's activities, ABA and other therapies, work, chores, relaxing, self-care, exercise, screen time, drinking alcohol, and sports are categories to look at.

Next, prioritize your categories in the same fashion you itemize your financial spending. Just like with your finances, where can you take time and place it toward activities that are supporting your functional medicine lifestyle? **Plan how you will make time for this lifestyle.**

Let's talk about Screen time! Have you ever calculated how much time you look at a screen at work and at home? Are you constantly looking at social media and what/who you follow? There are TV and video games. It adds up. Eyes become strained and focus is affected. This also impacts relationships. Even when talking to a family member, are they or are you looking at a screen? What else could you be doing other than screen time? A hobby, socializing, movement, self-care?

Finding Financial Freedom

Dave Ramsey's Financial Peace University is the best prerequisite for approaching the functional medicine process and partnership. Dave walks his audience through baby steps to pay off debt and build savings. His baby-step methodology is so similar to planning and implementing your functional medicine plan. You can find Financial Peace University community classes at his website ramseysolutions.com. He also offers a free budget resource called everydollar.com.

Schedule demands, finances and debt are *significant* sources of inflammation. Stress is inflammatory and disease- provoking. Remember, functional medicine is about the entire person and all facets of life.

So, How Do You Get the Most ROI (Return on Investment) From Your Functional Medicine Plan?

For functional medicine to be successful, you must have a plan of how you will make **time** to cook, **time** for stress management, **time** for self-care, **time** for relationships (not just driving your kids around), and how you will direct the **money** you do have toward your values and priorities.

Identify what you have space (time and money) for and find ways to direct these two currencies toward what you want.

At first you may think thoughts of what you can't do. Remember to first reach for better feeling thoughts by relying on the emotional scale, breath work, PARTS work, and create new key concepts/affirmations around time and money. This is how you shift your focus from what you can't do to identifying what you can do!

Decision-Balance

It's common to have mixed feelings when deciding to make a change. One thing that helps people when thinking of changing is to evaluate the pros and cons of their current behavior and the pros and cons of changing that behavior before making a final decision. The decision-balance exercise guides you to do a cost-benefit analysis about the change you are contemplating making.

Decision-making was conceptualized by Janis and Mann (1977) as a decisional "balance sheet" of comparative potential gains and losses. Two components of decisional balance, the pros, and the cons, have become core constructs in the Transtheoretical Model (TTM) (Prochaska & DiClemente, 1983; Prochaska, DiClemente, & Norcross, 1992)

In Chapter One you were introduced to the Stages of Change that are a part of the Transtheoretical Model (TTM). The five stages are **pre-contemplation** (not ready), **contemplation** (getting ready), **preparation** (ready), **action, and maintenance**. The TTM model teaches the decision-balance principle to reduce resistance, facilitate progress, and prevent relapse at various stages of the change process.

As individuals progress through the Stages of Change, decisional balance shifts in critical ways. When an individual is in the pre-contemplation stage, the pros in favor of behavior change are outweighed by the relative cons for change and in favor of maintaining the existing behavior. In the contemplation stage, the pros and cons tend to carry equal weight, leaving the individual ambivalent toward change. If the decisional balance is tipped, however, such that the pros in favor of changing outweigh the pros of maintaining the unhealthy behavior, many individuals move to the preparation or even action stage. As individuals enter the maintenance stage, the pros in favor of maintaining the behavior change should outweigh the cons of maintaining the change to decrease the risk of relapse.

Use the graph on the following page, to list in one place, the pros, and cons of changing and the pros, and cons of continuing your current behavior. Seeing the full array of pros and cons can make it easier to decide if you are ready to make the change (action). **Ask yourself if it is worth the cost to change? Is it worth the cost to stay the same?**

For example, list the **pros** of directing funds to functional medicine's out-of-pocket expenses. Then list the **cons** of directing funds to functional medicine.

List the **pros** of *not* directing money toward functional medicine. List the **cons** of *not* directing money toward functional medicine.

	Changing	Not Changing
Pros		
Cons		

Let's Talk About Functional Labs and Supplement Protocols

Our goal at Hope for Healing is to empower you, our patients, and community members, to have a voice in the development of your personalized care plan.

At your initial new patient appointment, your medical provider is going to see the big picture of where they need to investigate further with diagnostic labs. Some examples of the labs recommended at Hope for Healing are CIRS biomarkers, Tick-Borne Complete, Neural Zoomer, GI Map, Organic Acid Test (OAT), etcetera.

Here is an introduction to some labs Hope for Healing uses regularly:

- **CIRS Biomarkers:** These labs evaluate how your environment may be affecting your health and causing symptoms.

- **Tick-Borne Complete:** Assesses for tick-borne diseases such as Lyme disease, Bartonellosis, Babesiosis, and Anaplasmosis.

- **Neural Zoomer:** Assesses circulating autoantibodies in the bloodstream that attacks the brain, nerves, and blood-brain barrier. This helps to evaluate for PANS/PANDAS.

- **GI Map:** Evaluates for a multitude of bacterial, fungal, viral, and parasitic pathogens within someone's gut. It also evaluates the normal bacterial flora, enzyme balance, and overall gut health.

- **OAT Test:** The purpose of the Organic Acid Test is to evaluate a person's metabolic health. It evaluates vitamin and mineral levels, oxidative stress, and neurotransmitter levels.

If your intuition is saying the recommended labs feels like too much, instead of getting overwhelmed, get intentional. At Hope for Healing, we empower our patients to have a voice in the development of their ongoing care. If the number of labs or supplements ever feels overwhelming, please feel confident to communicate, with integrity, your hesitation to complete all these labs and functional therapies and incur a large financial commitment at this time.

It's okay to say you understand we need to eventually order these tests and layer in these therapies; however, which ones are a priority and which ones can be left for future consideration?

By now, you accept that there is no quick fix to reversing complex dis-ease conditions, so it's perfectly acceptable to be co-creating care plans that are a match to your current time and financial thresholds.

It's important to think ahead and know that each lab will have a protocol that includes an elaborate supplement regimen and possible complimentary functional therapies. With this in mind, remember to keep treatment plans reasonable.

Our goal for you is to feel empowered at each medical visit and ready to get to work co-creating a reasonable care plan that you feel confident implementing and sustaining. We want you to walk out the door feeling like yes! I can do this! If you are not in 100% agreement with the treatment care plan, your provider needs to know! I watch a lot of people not speak up while with the provider and then go home and cherry-pick what they think they can do and what they feel is essential. This breaks down the patient-provider partnership and deteriorates the effectiveness of the treatment plan.

Remember, your Genetics Wellness Blueprint provides the foundation for your treatment. Without knowing your genetics, your medical provider is handicapped. That's why we require genetics at Hope for Healing; this provides you the best possible outcome when another treatment plan is implemented.

Let's talk more about supplement regimens and the associated cost. The sticker price often shocks patients at check out. When patients are presented with the total amount, it can feel like it's not affordable. It's important to take a moment and do some simple math and calculate the cost of supplements per day. Generally, supplement protocols can be as inexpensive as three dollars a day.

As you continue to partner with your provider, remember to have clear communication about a plan that is a match to your time and financial thresholds. We understand you feel pressed for time when life has been so disrupted by the diagnosis, however, there is so much benefit to working within your time and financial thresholds. Working slowly, intentionally on one test and protocol, following the protocol as it is designed, will better prepare you for the next step in your treatment plan. This is a much more sustainable approach than doing too much, all at once, feeling overwhelmed, and then not returning for your follow-up appointments.

At each follow-up, please be mindful to inquire which supplements are to be continued and which can be discontinued. And track when you discontinue a supplement in your Personalized Medicine Care Planner. We will talk more about tracking your protocols in Chapter Four.

Planning Time to Stabilize Changes

Remember in Chapter One, we introduced that stabilization is an often-overlooked piece to a comprehensive care plan? You feel like you are in a race against time and want to do as much as you can as quickly as you can! The truth is you cannot heal if you are always accelerating toward what's next. Please celebrate where you are, acknowledge your short-term gains, and begin contemplating and preparing your next three-month care plan. Thinking and feeling goals are equally as important as action and maintenance.

Please consider, at the end of your three-month care plan, scheduling a week on your calendar to stabilize the changes you have made prior to layering in more changes. Practice fine-tuning changes you have made and fully integrate them into your life, mind, and heart.

Prioritize therapies which assists the body in shifting from sympathetic overdrive into predominantly the parasympathetic, "rest and digest," nervous system. Our culture has us locked in a chronic sympathetic state and as mentioned, healing is prevented when the nervous system is constantly in a state of fight-or-flight. To find a structural integration therapist trained in Craniosacral Therapy and Lymphatic Drainage, go to upledger.com and search for a practitioner in your area. Another alternative is to google a physical therapist that offers Visceral Manipulation.

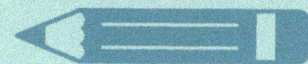

Being honest with yourself is the first step in genuine acceptance and a step closer to self-love. Just like your core, *clinical imbalances provide invaluable clues to what you can do to bring yourself back to balance, your thoughts also provide important insight into if you are helping or hindering healing.*

Where is your time going?

Do you have time to sustain ABA and other behavioral therapies and your functional medicine plan?

Prioritize the categories you spend your time:

Write your beliefs/thoughts/emotions around money in general and in relation to your health and well-being.

Do you have a family budget? Do you know where every dollar is going?

List where you think your money goes outside of your necessary bills. Think about eating out, fast food, coffees, memberships and subscriptions, clothes, entertainment, and alcohol. You may be surprised.

Explain how these itemized spending categories are supporting your functional medicine journey.

In what ways are you casting your time and money vote toward your health and well-being?

In what ways are you casting your time and money vote toward perpetuating your chronic condition?

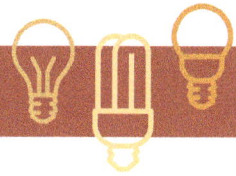

The Comprehension section is intended to optimize your comprehension. This section reviews the big ideas which make functional medicine provide the profound results we have come to expect. Think about what you have learned and how you will apply them to your unique and current circumstances.

Gut check your plan. Is it a match to your current time and financial thresholds?

What are you doing to find and address fixed mindsets around time and money?

What is your method for budgeting time and money toward your functional medicine journey?

What time and financial commitments are nurturing your functional medicine journey?

What time and financial commitments are sabotaging your financial medicine journey?

What resources will you use to work on finding financial freedom?

What steps are you taking to optimize your Return on Investment (ROI)?

Using the Decision-Balance what are the pros and cons of this new invest-ment portfolio?

How will you communicate feelings of financial overwhelm?

How will you plan for time to stabilize your changes before evolving your dynamic care plan?

Part 2: Communication and Interpersonal Skills to Build Better Relationships

In Chapter Two, Implement Your Plan!, you spent a lot of time working on your relationship with yourself and training your mind. The more you remove sources of inflammation, the more you train your mind and breathing, the better the relationship you have with yourself. Ultimately, you must become your own best coach. This will transfer to improving your relationships with those closest to you.

The Institute for Functional Medicine includes relationships as a modifiable lifestyle factor. Communication is essential in positive relationships.

How Do We Go "against the norm" Without Alienating Our Family, Inner Circle, and Work colleagues?

Are you familiar with **Nonviolent Communication (NVC)**? Expressing yourself through observation, feelings, needs, and requests without being too indirect and not being harmful to yourself and others. NVC is a communication skill that is incredibly useful in interpersonal relationships. positivepsychology.com/non-violent-communication/

You can find more resources to learn and apply NVC at the back of your workbook.

NVC is one way to practice communicating with your inner circle about your chosen changes. Another is to be cognizant of your word choices. **Our words can make a difference between polarizing or uniting us with our family, peers, your child's teachers, and your colleagues.** Your word choice could elicit *criticism or support* for your commitment to the functional medicine process. For example, notice the difference between the two statements.

"I'm on a restricted diet, so I can't eat that."

Or

"I am learning how certain foods create an inflammatory response, which aggravates my symptoms. I've started choosing foods that are low-inflammatory, to remove the burden and help heal the root causes of my symptoms. I'm really starting to feel the difference. Have you heard about high inflammatory foods?"

Two simple solutions to navigate family gatherings, social and work parties:

- Talk with the host ahead of time and share how you are learning how to heal the underlying sources creating your or your child's symptoms. Ask if you may bring a dish to a gathering. It's okay to ask permission if you may bring a small cooler so to be sure you have what you need.

- If you know which restaurant you will be attending, look at the menu ahead of time to see what options are available to you and maybe even call them to discuss certain menu items that look appealing to you. Then you are prepared to place your order with confidence and without drawing attention, if that is something you are concerned about.

We need to respect that our circle of family and friends are not making the same changes and may not understand why and what it really means to us.

Avoid oversharing your story and your care plan. This may not be useful.

Learning how to share your story in a way that's relatable and meaningful to the person you are talking to, so they don't only hear me, me, me is another thing to practice.

An Effective Structure to Share Your Story is-
"You know how (list a few pains associated with the diagnosis) really impact the quality of life? Well, I'm ready and willing to discover the root causes creating those symptoms rather than choosing to learn how to manage my symptoms with more band-aids. I'm learning about sources of inflammation. And since inflammation is at the root of all dis-ease, I'm taking steps to remove as much burden from my body as possible so I can (list what you hope to gain back into your life). When I talk about root cause medicine, what does that make you think about?"

Active Listening

Listening is the greatest communication skill anyone can develop. Listening has been shown to be essential to communicating respect for another person and is what builds trust and rapport. Active listening includes responses that demonstrate that you understand what the other person is trying to tell you about his or her experience and point of view. Active listening is a communication skill that involves going beyond simply hearing the words that another person speaks but also seeking to understand the meaning and intent behind them. It requires being an active participant in the communication process rather than just thinking about what you are going to say next. Developing active listening skills is a way to help diffuse strong emotional conversations and a tool to help people process complex information intertwined with decision-making.

When you share something, you are changing, this may ignite defensiveness in others because their preferences, habits, values, and character may feel threatened. Active listening is a skill to help you not take personally this defensiveness and will help you stay present for someone to give thought to their own change process. **Parents:** Active listening is one of the best parenting tools to add to your toolbox to reduce resistance to change and for conflict resolution.

Motivational interviewing is a counseling approach developed in part by clinical psychologists William R. Miller and Stephen Rollnick. It is a directive, client-centered counseling style for eliciting behavior change by helping clients to explore and resolve ambivalence. There are many books and videos to learn simple active listening skills such as *Motivational Interviewing with Adolescents and Young Adults* by Sylvie Naar and Mariann Suarez.

In brief, after the person has spoken, reflect back what you heard. This active listening technique ensures that you've captured the other person's thoughts, ideas, and/or emotions accurately. It also helps the other person feel validated and understood while keeping any potential miscommunications to a minimum.

One way to reflect what you've heard is to summarize. For example, you might say, "In other words, what you are saying is that you're frustrated because you don't know what diet lifestyle changes are right for you" or "I'm hearing that you're frustrated about the media villainizing gluten and dairy. Your Italian family has been eating gluten for centuries." Summarize what you heard and give the person the opportunity to say whether you've captured their meaning or intent. Think of yourself as a sounding board helping the other person articulate what's in their heart and on their mind.

People May Fall Out of Your Chosen Lifestyle: How Can You Be Okay With This?

This can be a tricky one and may need some skill to navigate and communicate. As you are changing your habits, activities, and lifestyle, you may find that those around you become distant. A divide appears and they may be upset and hostile that you are transforming and, in their eyes, moving away.

On the other side, you may decide you do not want to continue relationships that once served you, but do not anymore. This can cause stress and sadness. Remember, stress causes inflammation.

Drinking can bond people. Trauma can bond people. What's left when you are working on these things and no longer align with some people in your life?

"You are the average of the five people you spend the most time with." Jim Rohn

Counseling may become an important piece to your care plan to help you go through these big changes with those closest to you.

Character Strengths

Hopefully, you completed the VIA character strength survey and know your top five-character strengths. These can be used when communicating or finding the strength to communicate a difficult message. For example, some people rely on humor, while others rely on kindness or self-regulation.

Using character strengths and positive, nonviolent communication will be helpful. Asking permission to share information before doing so is also helpful. It's also acceptable to share the support that you like to receive and what that means to help you heal from the root causes creating your symptom set.

Remember to ask yourself if your words are *kind*, *true*, and *necessary*?

Communication with Your Hope for Healing Collaborative Care Team

At Hope for Healing, we recognize and honor the significance of healthy communication. It is only through healthy communication that our patients are not only best served by our entire team, but that we as the team are able to understand and participate in the health journey of our patients most effectively. For this reason, we ask that our patients agree to the superior communication standards outlined in the Memorandum of Understanding. We ask all patients to read the memorandum provided and signify your agreement by initialing next to each standard listed. The agreement is required to become a patient of our practice and failure to meet the agreed upon behavioral expectations may result in termination from the practice.

Our patients can expect to be treated with kindness, fairness, respect, and honesty. As a team, we hold ourselves to a superior standard in regard to customer service and patient care. It is our sole aim to communicate with complete empathy, courtesy, and a goal for resolution. We, therefore, hold our patients to a supreme standard as well, as it pertains to the treatment of our Hope for Healing providers and staff members. We too expect kindness, fairness, respect, and honesty from our patients. In matters of conflict or other arduous circumstances, we expect to be met with equal effort in working toward a resolution. This may involve compromise and will absolutely require proper appreciation and courtesy of all parties. To clarify and ensure necessary understanding, please review and initial the behavioral expectations outlined in the Memorandum of Understanding. We appreciate you agreeing to these communication standards when you that you agree to become a patient at Hope for Healing.

The comprehension section is intended to optimize your comprehension. This section reviews the big ideas which make functional medicine provide the profound results we have come to expect. Think about what you have learned and how you will apply them to your unique and current circumstances.

- **What skills have you learned to communicate with your inner circle regarding changes you are making?**

- **What does nonviolent communication mean to you and how will this affect your relationships?**

- **In what ways are you noticing and relying on your character strengths for effective communication?**

- **Communicating with the Hope for Healing Collaborative Care Team from a place of integrity means that I…. (complete the sentence)**

Chapter Three Summary

We have talked a lot about being an effective, equal therapeutic partner with your Collaborative Care Team. We recommend the perspective that you are partnering with those around you – your family, your child, educators, employers, friends, and colleagues – for the success of your hope for healing, functional medicine journey. Effective partnerships need well-defined roles and responsibilities, a budget for time and money, and effective communication! Communication, time, and money are the currencies you will use to sustain your path of transformation; therefore, I refer to them as your Functional Finances.

Build Your Personalized Care Plan

List the nutrition and lifestyle changes from Chapter One, the mental, emotional, and spiritual components you are using to implement your plan from Chapter Two, and the time, money, and communication steps you are willing to take from this week.

Supplement, Rx, Medical Protocols

Therapies | Structural Integration | Bodywork

Modifiable Lifestyle Factors

Mental | Emotional | Spiritual

Chapter Three Homework

Along with the obvious lifestyle factors of nutrition, movement, relationships, sleep, and stress reduction, *time*, *money, and effective communication* must be considerations. *Schedules, finances, and negative, aggressive communication are sources of inflammation.* Reducing the stress, worry, and uncertainty around time and money, as well as transforming your communication style, needs to be important considerations when creating, implementing, and sustaining your personalized care plan.

Journal prompts:

- **Financial Budget**: where is your money going?

  - What is your relationship with money?

  - How are you prioritizing funds toward your functional medicine journey?

  - Is this aligned with your values and beliefs and priorities?

  - What changes could you/are you ready to make?

  - Find a Dave Ramsey's Financial Peace University near you by visiting his website: ramseysolutions.com

- **Time Budget:** where are you spending your time?

  - Identify where you have time for your care plan action items.

  - Multi-tasking is a term used in computer programming. How can you multi-task less and focus more?

- What would it feel like to not try and accomplish so much on any given day?

- Are you planning for a time to stabilize your changes?

- **Communication**
  - What nonviolent communication techniques have you learned? And which ones have you practiced?

  - How can you use your character strengths?

  - Create an elevator pitch: A minute statement about why you are changing and "going against the norm" with diet and lifestyle choices.

    - This is what's going on (pain), and this is what I've learned is creating my pain and this is what I've decided to do about it to help me gain back *XYZ*. And here's how it's working (I'm experiencing more energy ...) Have you heard of functional medicine -root cause medicine?

  - How will you prepare to communicate and work with your Collaborative Care Team from a place of empowerment rather than emotional distress?

VERY IMPORTANT! Look ahead to Chapter Four and begin to write your story using the Care Plan Template. Next, please type your story from your care plan template and keep it to document your journey and prepare for your medical visits..

There is power in writing and speaking what is going well, writing about the better feeling thoughts you are training your mind to reach for each moment of your day, writing about your peaks and valleys, and the strengths you are relying on along the way!

This exercise is designed to prepare you to feel empowered in your initial new patient appointment and get right to work with your provider. The template organizes how you will share the personalized care plan you have been working on up until the initial appointment. You will discuss your perceived sources of inflammation (your health history timeline), how you are assuming responsibility for your nutrition and lifestyle modifications (autonomy), which changes you have successfully stabilized, and what you feel are the next changes to be layered in based on your current ability (motivation + confidence + competence). You are now ready to have a voice in the co-creation of the medical interventions to ensure they are a match to your emotional and financial threshold.

This exercise empowers you to be an active participant in your care as an equal, therapeutic partner with your medical provider. Based on your history, genetics, and lifestyle plan you share, your provider will fulfill their role and responsibilities by recommending the diagnostic labs to determine exactly the sources of inflammation to address first, supplements to give your body the necessary nutrients to function more effectively, perhaps any prescriptions, as well as functional therapies that may be appropriate and timed safely.

Chapter 4: Tell Your Story!

Key Terms

Visceral Manipulation: a hands-on therapy that focuses on your organs. The main area of focus is typically your abdomen. The goal is to relieve tension, improve connective tissue mobility, and encourage better digestive function.

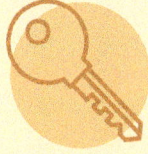

Gene-Environment Interaction: the interactions between genes and environment shape human development. Your genetic expression is largely determined by your nutrition and environment.

Safe Zone: reducing and eventually eliminating high-allergen, processed foods you bring into your home.

Genetic Wellness Blueprint: a genetic test panel used by Hope for Healing medical providers to steer personalized treatments.

Part 1: Review
- Acknowledge all the lessons learned that set you up for success.

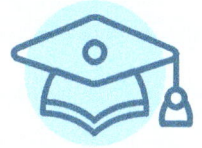

Part 2: The Environment is Everything
- The home is your healing headquarters.
- Create a safe zone.
- Focus on success habits.

Part 3: Tell Your Story!
- Meet your medical provider from a state of empowerment rather than emotional distress.
- Trust your medical provider.
- Be an inspiration to more people tired of managing symptoms with band-aids.

Introduction

In this chapter we review what we have learned, as well as discover how to create an atmosphere conducive to healing as you go through your change process and your hope for healing, functional medicine journey. You will be well-prepared and empowered to work with your medical team to reduce overwhelm, optimize outcomes, and tell your story to inspire more people who are thinking to pursue root-cause medicine.

Part 1: Review

What is Functional Medicine?

The future of medicine must be in the hands of the people, understanding how to take control of their health and transform their lives so they can live their most purpose-filled lives!

Functional medicine is the science of creating health. It is the medicine of "why." Functional medicine is patient-centered, not disease-centered. Your comprehensive care plan includes all facets of your well-being including finances, time, communication, mental, emotional, and spiritual components, nutrition, and lifestyle. Your health impacts all these facets and likewise, they all impact your health.

Equal, Therapeutic Partnership

Functional medicine is a mutual-participatory medical model where the patient and provider work as equal therapeutic partners. Each partner has a role and responsibilities.

Your role is implementation. Functional medicine's success is largely determined by how well the patient or parent can implement and layer pieces of a comprehensive care plan to work in combination and sustain the changes. Your responsibilities are to learn mind-body medicine, self-directed neuroplasticity, and breathing techniques, be accountable to budget your time and money, and practice nonviolent communication to build better relationships with yourself, family, friends, colleagues, community, and Hope for Healing's Collaborative Care Team. Additional responsibilities are to be prepared for your appointments, to keep your appointments, and to show up ready to get to work. This group coaching series is designed to establish clear, reasonable expectations so the partnership can be successful.

You Have Power in Your Outcome

Right now, life may feel like a living Hell. Living with a chronic condition and/or Autism, PANS, PANDAS takes us to the darkest, deepest levels of despair. Fortunately, we now know what is causing so much pain. It is no longer a mystery. You have a plan to move you in the direction of hope and healing. Your plan is reasonable and a match to your current ability. You have an entire team ready and willing to walk with you through your journey of transformation. You can do this! Trust the process and you will experience profound results.

What is Burdening Your or Your Child's Body and Mind?

Functional medicine is all about an inflammation hunt.

The functional medicine process can be summarized by the 5Rs: ***Remove, Replace, Reinoculate, Repair,*** and ***Rebalance.*** This group coaching has focused on the first two Rs, Remove and Replace, with the following:

- **Lifestyle:** (stress, habits, movement, sleep, relationships, time, finances, communication)—all the modifiable lifestyle factors.

- **Nutrition:** removing the high-allergens is truly a prerequisite before committing to working with a provider and is honestly how you optimize your results!

- **Stress & Resilience:** acknowledging emotional toxicity and emotional stress/trauma. Seeking support to discuss traumas, such as counseling, energy work, and structural integration therapies.

- **Implementing:** the mental and emotional facets of a comprehensive care plan. Applying self-directed neuroplasticity, and mind-body medicine techniques to reach for better feeling thoughts to guide your words, actions, habits, character, and destiny.

- **Sustaining:** planning to deliberately direct your time and money toward your functional medicine journey.

- **Communicating:** embracing nonviolent communication to build better relationships/partnerships.

The Comprehension section is intended to optimize your comprehension. This section reviews the big ideas which make functional medicine provide the profound results we have come to expect. Think about what you have learned and how you will apply them to your unique and current circumstances.

- **What does current ability mean to you?**

- **What change do you feel especially successful in?**

- **What are you relying on to feel successful?**

- **What are the four main initiators of inflammation?**

- **Based on your health history timeline, list three initiators you discovered over the course of this group coaching series.**

- **What key concept have you create regarding self-acceptance, and self-love.**

- What key concepts have you made to create new healthy thought patterns and beliefs?

- What are you celebrating?

- List three ways you are working to sustain your functional medicine journey.

- Yes or No, has there been a time that you used nonviolent communication skills in the last week to work with family members on resolving differences?

Part 2: The Environment is Everything

In this chapter, you apply all lessons learned to create an atmosphere that is conducive to healing. **Healing is done at home, not at therapy sessions or doctor's appointments. You or your child can do all the therapy and see all the doctors in the world, however, if the home atmosphere is moldy, stressed, disorganized, and chaotic, healing will be blocked.**

The environment in which we live, work, and interact with interplays with our genetic vulnerabilities. This combination is what sets the stage for patients to tip into certain disease states. When our environment is toxic (emotional stress, trauma, dietary stress, hidden pathogens, chemical/heavy metal/mold exposures, financial and time constraints, negative, aggressive communication) our genetic variants are adversely affected, and function is diminished.

The good news is that our environment, both internally and externally, is modifiable! You have great power in optimizing your outcomes. Since the environment is everything, let's take a look at our home environment and turn your home into your headquarters for healing.

Make a Safe Zone!

What does it mean to turn your home into your headquarters for healing?

If mold is suspected, that is the number one priority. Work with Hope for Healing to identify what you can do to remove yourself and safely remediate the mold.

Regarding nutrition and lifestyle changes, before changing your social life, it is recommended to **first start making your home a safe zone.** Work to reduce the amount of high-allergen, processed foods you bring into your home. Ultimately, work to not have any inflammatory foods in your headquarters. This is good for the entire family! We are bombarded with refined sugar products and processed foods everywhere! At first, let your exposures to these high-allergens be when you are outside your headquarters. Over time, the symptoms that occur from consuming high inflammatory food triggers will make the triggering foods less and less appealing. The high inflammatory foods will eventually become associated with pain rather than pleasure.

In addition to the dietary sources of inflammation being eradicated from your headquarters, also address the toxic common home goods exposures which are contributing to your inflammatory load. Reference the Menu of Nutrition and Lifestyle Options toward the back of your workbook. Use this menu to continuously evolve your care plan.

The EPA states our indoor air quality is more toxic than the outdoor air quality. How so? Chemicals! Only when we begin to pay attention, can we fully understand the number of toxic substances we are exposed to each day, many of which are neurotoxins. Consider this list and begin to investigate the toxicity of common household items. To evaluate common household items, use the Environmental Working Group EWG's Healthy Living app or Think Dirty app for personal care products. These apps are an easy way to learn about the potentially toxic ingredients in common products such as

- Skincare/makeup
- Cleaning products
- Carpets (VOCs, volatile organic compounds)
- Air fresheners (think Glade Plug-In)
- Nonstick cookware
- Unpurified water
- Plastic
- Perfumes
- Exposure to chemicals and heavy metals in the food/air/water

You don't need to throw out all food, cleaning products, or personal care products. This could lead to a big expense. As you use items, *replace* them with cleaner, natural, and toxin/chemical-free options. Start visiting farmers' markets or CSAs (community supported agriculture) for organic produce at a reasonable price and maybe do a little research on natural methods of cleaning your home. For example, I love using baking soda and white vinegar for cleaning. Needs a little bit of elbow grease, but isn't that a form of movement?

Communication sets the tone of the home atmosphere! Remember Chapter Two and Three! Continuously train your mind to reach for better feeling thoughts and speak words of hope and healing to yourself, to your family, and throughout your home. If you need to vent to a friend or family member, please do so when no children are around. Even our children with Autism can understand what we are saying even if it looks like they are not paying attention. Working on your communication styles with yourself and others is a must to create an atmosphere conducive to healing.

Place more focus on returning joy to your home than on the fear and adversity of a complex medical condition.

Bringing it all Home!

Use your training from Chapter Two and practice being mindful of the words you speak. Remember to ask yourself if the words you use are true, kind, and necessary? Make it a priority to talk about your family's accomplishments to your child, and to your family members. Tell them what great things you are all doing together and how you are feeling really good and encouraged about the journey you are on with Hope for Healing. Thank your children for teaching you what you need to do to help everyone feel better. **Be intentional to *elevate the good*.**

Remind yourself and your child that the diagnosis does not define you. You are so much more than just a collection of symptoms. The symptoms are communication that you or your child need to reduce inflammation and provide beneficial nutrients to assist the body to move back toward homeostasis/balance! You can reassure your family by saying *"This is just something we are moving through. We have an entire team helping us resolve what is causing us pain. We've got this. We are learning all the things we can do as a family to help us feel better! And when we feel better, we can have way more fun!"*

This is an example of speaking healing words over your family that create an atmosphere conducive to healing!

Part 3: Tell Your Story!

Tunnel Vision

Please take a moment and reflect on the last six weeks of accomplishments. Look for small things that have improved. It is common to have tunnel vision when living with a challenging health diagnosis. Patients often overlook aspects that have improved because so many symptoms remain. The eighth-week mark is usually when small improvements appear if you are looking for them!

You have written your perceived sources of inflammation (your health history timeline), how you are assuming responsibility for your nutrition and lifestyle modifications (autonomy), which changes you have successfully stabilized and what you feel are the next changes to be layered in based on your current ability (motivation + confidence + competence).

Remember: This exercise is designed to prepare you to feel empowered in your initial new patient appointment and get right to work with your provider. The template organizes how you will share the personalized care plan you have been working on up until the initial appointment.

Care Plan Template

I sought out functional medicine because _____ (motivators)

My top three concerns are _____

_____

_____

_____

I desire to gain back _____

_____

_____

_____

_____ into my life as a result of my functional medicine journey.

Functional medicine means _____

_____

_____

_____

_____ to me.

I've learned from my health history timeline that my family history of _____

_____

_____

_____

_____ and my triggering emotional stress and traumas such as

_____

_____

_____

____ have been antecedents and/or mediators in my development of symptoms.

And my ongoing exposures to the following dietary, lifestyle, chemicals/heavy metals/mold such as _____

_____

_____

_____

_____ have interacted with my genetic variants to manifest my symptom set.

I understand I have these SNPs that are relevant to the following systems of my body: *(If you are waiting for your genetic results or delaying them until you are financially prepared, then please complete this section later.)*

- Improving brain function:

  _____

  _____

  _____

- Decreasing inflammation:

  _____

  _____

  _____

- Improving autophagy:

  _____

  _____

  _____

- Improving vitamin B12 delivery:

  _____

  _____

  _____

- Improving methylation:

  _____

  _____

  _____

- Improving mitochondrial function:

  _____

  _____

  _____

I have these questions about my genetics:

_____

_____

_____

These are the nutrition and lifestyle changes I've successfully implemented and stabilized prior to this appointment:

_____

_____

_____

I chose these first because they were in my current ability. A few things that I relied on to successfully change are *(Think breaking down into small steps, support, character strengths, inspiration, accountability, measuring goals, etcetera)*:

_____

_____

_____

I'm inspired to layer in these next modifiable nutrition and lifestyle changes:

_____

_____

_____

I feel I need this support to assist me with my self-acceptance and continued change process

_____

_____

_____

A few *"aha moments"* I had through this process of preparing to layer on the genetic and medical pieces to my comprehensive care plan were:

_____

_____

_____

I understand that insurance does not accept functional medicine and that it's up to me to understand medical costs and drive health care decisions with you as an equal partner. If recommendations feel overwhelming, is it ok if I ask which ones are priority and which can be left for future considerations?

I understand that nonviolent communication with my Collaborative Care team is a value I agree with.

In addition, I would like to share this:

_____

_____

_____

Preparing for Follow-up Visits

This series has walked you through designing a nutrition and lifestyle plan based on your current ability, strategies to implement your plan, sustain your plan, and communicate your plan.

The follow-up appointments are targeted reviews based on your last appointment, however, there may be additional concerns you would like to address. In order to prepare for follow-up appointments, you will be completing forms before each follow-up appointment. Please communicate prior to your follow-up visits if your child will *not* be present.

Be ready to communicate your main concerns. Your provider will let you know which ones are relevant to the purpose of the follow-up and what are the next steps for addressing the remaining concerns at the next scheduled follow-up appointment. **Also, at the start of your follow-up appointments, ask if the provider will update which supplements to continue and which can be discontinued. Be sure to document this in your Personalized Medicine Care Planner.**

Next Steps!
Genetics

Ideally, genetics come next to have an insight into your genetic predispositions. Without genetics, we are all flying blind. Genetic testing provides you with evidence-based, personalized action steps based on your unique biological makeup to ensure that any recommendations made are both necessary and effective. Genetics is the missing puzzle piece in the medical mystery cases of many patients, the guide to preventative care, and a key tool for those seeking to optimize their health and performance.

This is when you really start knowing how to work with your body rather than against it.

Your genes are not your destiny. Since your genetic expression largely is determined by your environment, and your environment is modifiable, the lifestyle changes you are implementing will interact with your SNPs (single nucleotide polymorphisms) for favorable outcomes.

Additionally, the genetic testing we offer provides insight into hard-wired, non-epi-genetically modifiable SNPs. Some supplements and medications you must take forever because your body cannot make the necessary enzymes to decrease inflammation, detoxify/clean out your cells, increase your brain regenerative capacity, improve neurologic function, and give your body more energy.

We need to understand your genetic vulnerabilities and then know the precise lifestyle/nutrition/supplements your body's blueprint requires to regain balance. To learn more about Hope for Healing's Genetic Care Path, visit get2theroot.com and schedule a Genetics Orientation. Hope for Healing uses a Wellness Blueprint genetic panel that is a cheek swab.

Ongoing Coaching

Having a guide, who knows this journey well, is invaluable. Mastering nutrition and lifestyle changes is a constant evolution. Continuing with coaching packages is an affordable and effective way to make sure you continually convert the initial boost of enthusiasm into endurance for your functional medicine journey. Coaches support you in bridging the gap between knowing what needs to be done and doing what needs to be done. This includes everything from making your next appointment to implementing a treatment plan.

Medical: Initial New Patient Visit

The external environment affects your genes and your internal environment. The hidden sources of inflammation of gut and body pathogens (bacteria, viral load, parasites) and toxicity need to be identified through medical diagnostics ordered by your functional medicine provider. This is when you get into the remaining three Rs: **Reinoculate**, **Repair**, and **Rebalance**. Please partner with your provider to co-create a reasonable plan. Remember, when you walk out the door the goal is for you to feel like yes! I can do this! Please trust your providers' guidance. If there's something you are uncomfortable with or feel overwhelmed, your provider needs to know. At the end of the visit, please have a plan that both you and your provider agree on.

This is just the beginning …

We highly encourage you to continue writing and telling your story! Individuals like yourself are changing the face of healthcare in America.

When you're ready to share your story with others, I highly recommend working with my publisher, Braughler Books. Their mission is helping people tell their stories — and they have helped hundreds of authors do that over the years, just as they helped me. For more information, visit BraughlerBooks.com.

You have identified sources of inspiration for yourself as you travel this functional medicine journey. It's time now to remember that your story can be an inspiration for others.

At first, people will ask why you are doing it. Then they will ask you how you did it!

Menu of Nutrition and Lifestyle Options

Your health is largely determined by your nutrition, stress, environment, and genetic code. Nutrition and lifestyle changes are how you unlock your greatest potential.

Use these nutrition and lifestyle modifications like a menu. Select the ones that feel easy and within your current ability. Get excited about the basics and over time you will be able to add in changes that at one time felt impossible. If you place priority on the basics, you allow the more sophisticated medical interventions to provide significant results.

Any of these menu options in and of themselves will not cure nor will they fix any developmental/chronic/degenerative condition. However, when you begin to investigate the hidden sources of inflammation, hopefully, you will decide you want to do what you can to reduce and remove exposure to harmful chemicals and foods that are causing inflammation and pain. When you choose to remove harmful chemicals and processed foods from your life, consider the impact this also has on our environment. The way you spend your time and money is how you cast your vote for the kind of world you wish to live in.

"Master the Basics" is a good motto. Mastering the basic nutrition and lifestyle changes is the secret to getting the best return on investment from your functional medicine journey. There is also a medical section to prepare you for topics you may be talking about with your medical provider.

Stress & Resilience Modifications

Even with so much technology that supposedly makes our lives easier, the epidemic of stress is at an all-time high. It's common to feel as though more and more demands continue to bury us until we feel suffocated, choking, gasping for air, crushed.

The stress interacting with your genetic vulnerabilities can easily tip you into unhealthy coping strategies such as lack of sleep, overeating, drinking in excess, and other reward-seeking behaviors.

Since stress affects our sleep, that means it affects our cortisol and adrenal glands. When the adrenal glands start to collapse, we often see a domino effect with the gastrointestinal and detoxification systems. Then, we are stressed, tired, and sick!

Time and Money: Direct your time and money toward your investment in YOU and your family's health and well-being. This is how you truly cast your vote in this world. Health is a continuum. At all times we are either moving away or toward well-being.

Lymphatic Drainage: Your lymphatic system is the system responsible for eliminating cellular waste products. When your lymphatic system is not working properly, waste and toxins can build up and make you sick. Lymphatic congestion is a major factor leading to inflammation and disease. By gently stimulating your lymphatic system, it helps it release toxins. Lymphatic massage, jumping on a trampoline, and dry-skin brushing are powerful detoxification aids.

Stretching: When we're stressed not only does our heart rate increase but we tend to tighten our muscles. The benefits of stretching are many, such as stress relief, flexibility, improved posture (which helps to alleviate back pain), better sleep, injury prevention, prepares the body for exercise, and helps to enhance mental clarity.

Yoga: Yoga has many styles, forms, and intensities. Choose a class and an instructor wisely based on your, you guessed it, current ability! Numerous studies have shown that yoga may help reduce stress and anxiety. Yoga can enhance your mood and overall sense of well-being. Research Yoga Nidra.

Mediation Apps: Meditation apps are useful to help make meditation easier and more intuitive. Apps such as: Calm, Insight Timer, Headspace Meditation & Sleep, Ten Percent Happier Meditation, Buddhify, Unplug, and Simple Habit.

Pilates: Pilates is a type of mind-body exercise developed in the early twentieth century by Joseph Pilates.

Journaling: Write exactly how you are feeling. Express all the heartache and horror you feel. Then use the Emotional Scale to incrementally work your way up to a better feeling thought. It's okay to feel lousy and down. These mood behaviors can improve as you balance your physiological systems! While you are healing, it's best to not linger too long in lower fear-based thoughts. We must be constantly training our minds. Feeling joy is an incremental process. You can't get to joy from depression or anger; you must incrementally work your way toward a sense of joy and freedom. All the action won't do anything if you feel depressed about what actions you are doing.

Breathing Techniques: Being conscious and breathing fully can lead to deep relaxation, decreased pain, and improved mental state. Read about deep abdominal breathing and practice the segmented breathing exercise regularly. Notice throughout your day if you are holding your breath, which most of us do when we are in sympathetic nervous system overdrive (fight, flight, freeze, or fear). The Breathing Prayer and 4-7-8 Breathing exercises in Chapter Two are other exercises that help ground you and move you into parasympathetic nervous system rest and digest.

Hobbies: Hobbies can be a rewarding and satisfying way to lead a fuller and healthier life, and they can lead to an increased sense of well-being. How can you make even a small amount of time directed toward something you enjoy, toward a playful, engaging activity? This goes back to your time modifiable lifestyle change.

Essential Oils: With chronic diseases and developmental diagnosis, you may encounter challenges daily, such as anger, anxiety, meltdowns, insomnia, poor focus, muscle tension, and overall stress. When choosing essential oils, consider an organic, small essential oil business rather than an MLM. http://Chakrabalanceshop.com created a 7-month Subscription Box dedicated to assisting with your guided strategic sequence of the Hope for Healing Workbook.

Earthing: Get outside!!! Earthing (also known as grounding) refers to the discovery that bodily contact with the Earth's natural electric charge stabilizes physiology at the deepest levels, reduces inflammation, pain, and stress, improves blood flow, energy, and sleep, and generates greater well-being.

Nutrition Modifications

Food is information, not just energy (calories). Food tells your body how to function by signaling exactly when and how each different type of cell should behave in every situation.

A properly functioning digestive system is critical to you enjoying good health. In fact, problems with the gastrointestinal (GI) tract can cause more than just stomach aches, gas, bloating, or diarrhea.

GI issues may underlie chronic health problems that seem unrelated to digestive health, including autoimmune diseases such as rheumatoid arthritis and Type 1 diabetes, skin problems such as eczema, acne, and rosacea, heart disease, asthma, cognitive decline symptoms such as brain fog, depression, focus, anxiety, and Autism (just to name a few).

You are now familiar with Functional Medicine's 5Rs: Remove, Replace, Reinoculate, Repair, and Rebalance.

1. **Remove:** Remove stressors. Get rid of things that negatively affect the environment of the GI tract including high-allergen foods to start.

2. **Replace:** Replace with low inflammatory nutrition and non-toxic household items. Replace digestive secretions. Add back things like digestive enzymes, hydrochloric acid, and bile acids that are required for proper digestion under a medical provider's supervision.

3. **Reinoculate:** Help beneficial bacteria nourish by ingesting probiotic foods or supplements that contain the "good" GI bacteria such as Bifidobacteria and Lactobacillus species, and by consuming the high-soluble fiber foods that good bugs like to eat, called prebiotics.

4. **Repair:** Help the lining of the GI tract repair.

5. **Rebalance:** It is important to pay attention to lifestyle choices. Sleep, exercise, and stress can all affect the GI tract. Balancing those activities is important to an optimal digestive tract.

What is a Leaky Gut?

Leaky gut is *all* about the GALT and the gut. GALT stands for **g**ut **a**ssociated **l**ymphoid **t**issue. That's where immune activation, inflammation control, and healing take place. The GALT is actually a portion of the immune system located in the gut. Actually, 70 percent of immune tissue is in the small intestine and determines a profound amount of our total immune response. This is where nasty invaders like bacteria can be stopped before entering into circulation or paradoxically our gut can think we are being invaded with a "leaky gut" and mount an immune response (unnecessarily) to the food we eat. Gluten and other high-allergen foods cause damage and open holes in the gut. Simplistically speaking, gliadin (a substance within gluten) then gets through the cracks and leaks into your system and, contributes to the leaky gut syndrome. It also contributes to inflammation. An overactive immune response is triggered as your body tries to attack the foreign invader, in this case, gliadin (from gluten). You need healthy bacteria to properly digest gluten, casein, soy, and corn. Antibiotics, which many people have taken in abundance, kill bacteria, even the good kind in your gut.

This, then, affects one's ability to digest gluten and the other high-allergen foods. Toxins of many kinds can also increase intestinal permeability as well as gut pathogens such as yeast, parasites, and bacteria. Nutritional deficiencies, poor digestion, and the Standard American Diet high in inflammatory, processed foods also contribute to a gut becoming leaky. Most of the factors that increase intestinal permeability can be treated and, therefore, our food allergies, food sensitivities, and chronic symptoms can be lessened, and our health can be greatly improved. By being committed to consistently replacing offending food, you allow the leaky gut to be healed and more foods will become tolerated over time.

Changing food habits can be a complex, difficult, and sometimes confusing process. There are recipes, snack suggestions, a shopping list, and other information to make this more reasonable. Remember to use lessons learned in Chapter Two to help you remain focused on your plan rather than all the seemingly insurmountable obstacles.

What happened to Gluten?: Historically, wheat had been 97 percent starch, and 3 percent protein. By the 1870s, hybridized wheat had been introduced, a wheat with a protein content of 26 percent compared to the 3 percent it was previously. That's almost a 900 percent increase in the amount of gluten. This "super-wheat" made for better-baked goods for the American palate. But it also made for leaky guts! And allergic reactions!

Why No Gluten?: Gluten causes damage and opens the holes in the gut. Gliadin (from gluten) then gets through the cracks and leaks into your system, which is "leaky gut" and causes inflammation. Then there's an overactive immune response as your body tries to kill the foreign invader, in this case, gliadin. In order to heal the gut and stabilize your immune response, high-allergen foods must be removed.

Hidden Sources of Gluten: Soy sauce, caramel coloring, and artificial flavors on a food label almost certainly have gluten. Ask your coach about hidden sources of gluten.

Gluten-Free Crap Trap: Processed food is processed—even if it's gluten-free. The goal is to move toward whole foods, not replace processed foods with packaged gluten-free foods. Use these sparingly.

Dairy: Dairy, like gluten, is very hard to break down. Dairy is homogenized and pasteurized, which breaks protein down into inflammatory molecules. It makes for inflammatory milk! Casein, contained within dairy products, is gluten cross-reactive and inflammatory. At Hope for Healing, we do not recommend dairy products except for grass-fed organic butter or ghee.

High-Allergen Foods: Top food allergens: gluten, dairy, corn, eggs, soy, nuts, nightshades (tomatoes, bell peppers, potatoes, and eggplant), and sugar. Work to reduce exposure and crowd these out with other options.

Remove Food Dyes: Food dyes, synthesized originally from coal tar and now petroleum, have long been controversial because of safety concerns.

MSG: Friends don't let friends eat MSG. Monosodium glutamate is an excitotoxin and causes agitation, anxiety, fear, and a myriad of health problems.

NO GMO: Banned or restricted in over sixty countries. GMO stands for genetically modified organisms. GMOs are made by forcing genes from one species into the DNA of an unrelated species in order to introduce a new trait. This cannot occur in the natural world.

Antibacterial Soap: Concerns include whether these biocides are more effective than regular soaps, whether they may create new drug-resistant bacteria, and whether they may also act as hormone disruptors in humans or the environment.

Cookware: Remove toxic aluminum, and nonstick and replace with cast iron with or without enamel, stainless steel, or glass.

Remove Plastic: Remove plastic drinking cups and food storage containers and replace them with glass. Bottled water from plastic bottles contains phthalates or bisphenol A (BPA), which are toxic petrochemicals.

Diet to Regular Soda: Aspartame is a widely used artificial sweetener that has been linked to migraines. Upon ingestion, aspartame is broken, converted, and oxidized into formaldehyde in various tissues. At Hope for Healing, we do not recommend any type of soda, but as you are moving toward the elimination of soda, moving from diet to regular "sugary" soda is a better choice.

Glyphosate: Dr. Stephanie Seneff from the Massachusetts Institute of Technology (MIT) research has led her to the almost undeniable conclusion that glyphosate, the main ingredient in Roundup, is a major driver of autism and chronic conditions.

Food Chemicals: Packaged foods contain these synthetic flavoring chemicals which have been artificially made by flavor manufacturing engineers. The chemicals trick your mind to wanting more of the food. Ever wonder why you can't eat just one chip? It's important to read about excitotoxins.

Artificial Sweeteners: Choose the real thing, maple syrup, or local raw honey. Many published papers in PubMed say the overall use of artificial sweeteners remains controversial, and consumers should be amply informed about the potential risks of using them.

Smoothies with Benefits: Place in blender: 2 tablespoons flax seeds, 2 tablespoons protein powder, 1-2 cups whole vegetables, 1/2 cups fruit, and 4-6 ounces of base like coconut water, coconut milk, or tea (Pique Tea, mycotoxin/heavy metal-free).

Dining Out: Look ahead and determine what is available when you arrive at the restaurant. Bring your own toasted gluten-free buns for hamburgers and your own oil and vinegar for salad dressing. You're in luck! It's easier than ever to eat out and stay true to your low inflammatory style of eating.

No Nuts!: Tree nuts are one of the top allergens and most common food sensitivities. People with autoimmune diseases are very likely to have a leaky gut, which increases their susceptibility to developing food allergies and food sensitivities. If you find you are sensitive to nuts, use these helpful resources: Againstallgrain.com, Paleoplan.com, and thepaleomom.com (a note about Paleo—Paleo is high in saturated fat. At your genetic consult, be sure to ask about your ability to metabolize saturated fat.) If you have SNPs that affect the saturated fat response, you will want to modify Paleo recipes (don't rely on coconut oil for example!).

Stay Hydrated: Every day, drink approximately half your body weight in ounces of water and other non-caffeinated beverages free of added sugars.

Healthy Fats: Polyunsaturated fats from soybean, canola, and other seed oils are inflammatory. Choose ghee, duck fat, coconut oil, or avocado oil for high heat; drizzle olive oil on foods after they are cooked and use for salads. Coconut oil and avocado oil are good for baking.

Anti-Inflammatory Foods: Start by adding in the anti-inflammatory foods to start crowding out the more processed foods. The evidence is clear that such anti-inflammatory foods can regulate the immune system and impact the way inflammation affects our bodies and our lives. The darker the vegetable the higher the fiber content. Added bonus! Leafy greens, beets, bone broth, a palm-full of walnuts, ginger, bok choy, broccoli, wild salmon, chia seeds, freshly ground flax seeds, celery, blueberries, coconut oil, and turmeric are anti-inflammatory. (A note about flax seeds—they are high in oil and can go rancid quickly. Store in your freezer.)

Clean Fifteen. Dirty Dozen: A shopper's guide to pesticides in produce. Avoid the Dirty Dozen, the non-organic fruits, and vegetables that are highest in pesticide residues—and save money by choosing non-organic items from the Clean Fifteen list. Download the shopping guide from EWG.ORG to reduce your exposure to pesticides.

Clean 15	Dirty Dozen
Avocado	Strawberries
Sweet Corn	Spinach
Pineapple	Nectarines
Cabbage	Apples
Onion	Grapes
Frozen Sweet Peas	Peaches
Papaya	Cherries
Asparagus	Pears
Mango	Tomatoes
Eggplant	Celery
Honeydew Melon	Potatoes
Kiwi	Sweet bell peppers
Cantaloupe	
Cauliflower	
Broccoli	

Core or PhytoNutrient Food Plan: Ask about the Institute of Functional Medicine Core Food Plan or PhytoNutrient Food Plan. These food plans are helpful when transitioning to eating a whole-food diet.

Elimination Diet: High-allergen foods are removed for a full six weeks. The Elimination Diet helps to uncover food(s) that may be the culprits of pain. It is a very useful tool for diagnosing adverse food reactions, whether a true allergy, intolerance, or sensitivity. When you reintroduce a top food allergen, do so one at a time and eat it at least two to three times a day for three days to see if you notice a reaction. If you do, note the food, and eliminate it for ninety days or going forward. There are many Elimination Diet cookbooks. I like to think of this food plan as eliminating symptoms. Ask your health coach for the Institute of Functional Medicine's Elimination Diet food plan.

The two-page Elimination Diet Food Plan is designed to provide a snapshot of the foods that would be available to choose from every day.

Nutrition Plans

There are many fantastic resources today to help remove and replace high-allergen foods. Talk with your coach and medical providers about what's best for you and where to start. You can use these food plans as guidelines and as a resource for recipes.

The Institute for Functional Medicine has several food plans to talk about with your medical provider.

- Core Food Plan
- Phytonutrient Food Plan
- Elimination Diet
- Mito Food Plan
- Detox Food Plan
- FODMAPs
- Renew Food Plan

The Autoimmune Protocol (AIP) is a very restrictive diet that removes foods considered to be gut irritants. The AIP is a stricter version of the Paleo diet, which involves the elimination of grains, legumes, dairy, and processed foods.

The Specific Carbohydrate Diet (SCD) is a nutritionally complete grain-free diet, low in sugar and lactose. It was developed by Dr. Sidney Haas, a pediatrician in the 1920s, as a treatment for celiac disease and is used for other bowel disorders like ulcerative colitis and Crohn's disease.

Some families like a plan to follow such as the Autoimmune Protocol or Specific Carbohydrate Diet. Other families like to go much more slowly and work on replacing one offending food at a time, such as dairy, then gluten.

The Mito Food Plan

The Mito Food Plan may be described as an anti-inflammatory, low-glycemic, gluten-free, low-grain, high-quality fats approach to eating.

After you have worked with the Core Food Plan and possibly the Elimination Diet, another nutrition plan guideline to inquire about is the Mito Food Plan. This is an excellent plan to follow for Autism and other neurological conditions (like MS, Alzheimer's, and cognitive decline).

The plan focuses on supporting healthy mitochondria through the use of therapeutic foods that improve energy production. Mitochondria are structures in every cell that make energy by using oxygen and nutrients from food. The cells in the brain, heart, nerves, muscles, and organs all have higher concentrations of mitochondria. These parts of the body are also more susceptible to a premature decline in function caused by a host of common insults. Harmful food choices can contribute to this decline, leading to poor health and chronic illness. The Mito Food Plan will support the body in the production of energy, restore a sense of vitality, and help the body use food to support a graceful and healthy aging process.

Research has shown that diet and lifestyle interventions can be helpful in providing support for healthy mitochondria. When the mitochondria are working well, they help to reduce fatigue, pain, and cognitive problems while supporting muscle mass and burning excess fat.

As discussed above, the Mito Food Plan includes those foods that are known to support healthy mitochondrial function while maintaining blood sugar and inflammatory balance. The Mito Food Plan is from The Institute of Functional Medicine.

FODMAPs

Dr. Peter Gibson and Dr. Sue Shepherd
Certain types of carbohydrates often prove to be more challenging to digest. The unusual name FODMAP is an acronym for:

- **Fermentable**
- **Oligosaccharides**: carbohydrates which have three to ten simple sugars linked together, e.g., onions, garlic, leeks
- **Disaccharides**: lactose, sucrose, maltose
- **Monosaccharides**: a simple carbohydrate and a simple sugar. The molecules cannot be broken down (e.g excess fructose and glucose).
- **Polyols**: sugar-free sweeteners. They are carbohydrates but not sugar. They are used cup for cup to replace sugar. Some polyols are sorbitol, and mannitol.

Basically, FODMAPs are types of carbohydrates including sugars and fiber that are commonly found in many different types of food. These FODMAPs are difficult to digest in the small intestine, which is where the majority of the nutrients are absorbed in our body, so they sit here and end up feeding the microbes that live in the gut. These microbes include fungi and bad bacteria. This results in a fermentation process, which is responsible for those unpleasant, all too common symptoms such as flatulence, bloating, and belching.

Another side effect of these FODMAPS remaining in the colon is that they draw water to them which continues to perpetuate the bloating as well as adding cramping and potential constipation or diarrhea.

Food Group	Low FODMAP	High FODMAP
Dairy	Coconut milk, almond milk, oat milk	Most milks, most yogurts, cream, ice cream, sour cream
Proteins	Poultry, eggs, fish, beef, firm tofu, almonds	Soybeans, black beans, kidney beans, cashew nuts, silken tofu
Fruits	Oranges, lemons, limes, kiwi fruit, strawberries, bananas, blueberries	Apples, pears, plums, peaches, nectarines, watermelon
Vegetables	Tomato, zucchini, carrots, eggplant, potatoes	Corn, beets, sugar snap peas, asparagus, onion, garlic, mushrooms
Sweeteners	Maple syrup, stevia	High-fructose corn syrup, mannitol, sorbitol, honey

The idea of a low FODMAP diet is not to permanently remove all foods that are high in FODMAPS, because many of these provide fantastic nutrients that are essential to good health.

It's recommended to follow the FODMAP diet for eight weeks. After two months, other foods are reintroduced, one at a time. Documentation is key, helping you determine which foods work well and which foods cause a bad reaction in your body.

Lifestyle Modifications

Make Your Home a Safe Zone.

According to a *New York Times* article, many Americans assume that the chemicals in their shampoos, detergents, and other consumer products have been thoroughly tested and proven to be safe.

This assumption is wrong.

The Environmental Working Group conducted a study that shows the average newborn has 287 chemicals in the umbilical cord blood, 217 of which are neurotoxic. They include pesticides, phthalates, bisphenol A, flame retardants, and heavy metals such as mercury, lead, and arsenic.

The CDC says, in the last several years, a growing body of scientific evidence has indicated that the air within homes and other buildings can be more seriously polluted than the outdoor air in even the largest and most industrialized cities.

EWG's Healthy Living Home Guide

https://www.ewg.org/healthyhomeguide/

Water Filters: toxins like microbes, pesticides, plastics, prescription meds, metals, chlorine, fluoride, and others are poisoning our water supply. The Big Berkey and Aqua Tru are countertop filters. Aquasana offers whole-house water filtration units that are affordable. You may ozonate your water, too, to literally kill pathogens. Dr K recommends the promolife.com ozone generator.

The Scent of Danger: the Environmental Working Group (EWG) reports that while many popular perfumes, colognes, and body sprays contain trace amounts of natural essences, they also typically contain a dozen or more potentially hazardous synthetic chemicals, some of which are derived from petroleum and are known to be associated with hormone disruption and allergic reactions.

Mattresses: look for mattresses that have no less than 95 percent certified organic content. No polyurethane foam. No added chemical flame retardants [check baby mattresses!]. Look for low-VOC certification. No added fragrances or antimicrobials.

Flooring: use solid surface flooring instead of carpet. Choose FSC-certified solid wood (Forest Stewardship Council. Use natural linoleum or tile made in the US. Choose low-VOC finishes and sealants. Look for NSF-certified products. Install without glue; use nail-down or click lock. Avoid laminate, vinyl flooring, and synthetic carpeting. Read more at EWG.ORG

Flame-Retardant Materials: flame-retardant materials are in *everything*, especially baby mattresses, clothes, and anything cloth. Please learn about the chemicals in the retardant materials. Hopefully, you will feel inspired to choose natural fibers and non-toxic mattresses and furniture.

Air Filters: a report from the American Lung Association, with help from the Environmental Protection Agency, identified air toxicity as one of the top five most urgent environmental risks to public health.

Dr. K recommends purchasing either a whole-home air purifier called the Nano Induct or a Reme Halo. Also, consider purchasing a 250-square-foot personal iAdaptAir to take with you when you travel because it has a HEPA filter, ultraviolet light, and an ionization component. Go to https://www.airoasis.com/ and use the following discount code: *GET2THEROOT*

Mold: mold exposure causes a variety of health problems like brain fog, headaches, asthma, fatigue, insomnia, nausea, hair loss, hormonal imbalances, and autoimmunity, to name a few.

There are tests you can take and labs you can use to determine your exposure to mold toxins. They include the ERMI test from Envirobiomics and Mycometrics labs. The HERTSMI-2 test is a less expensive, but not as comprehensive test to determine if your home is a safe place to live or not. Hope for Healing carries these tests in the office. Please ask for them, if desired.

Household Cleaners: Environmental Workers Group (EWG's) Guide to Healthy Cleaning reviews and rates more than 2,000 popular household cleaning products with grades A through F, based on the safety of their ingredients and the information they disclose about their contents. Check ewg.org/guides/cleaners and see how your current cleaning supplies rate on their toxicity scale.

Dr. K recommends these resources for homemade cleaning products:

- DIY natural household cleaners by Matt and Betsy Jabs at diynatural.com
- *The Autoimmune Fix* by Dr. Tom O'Bryan has homemade cleaning solutions in the back of this book (pages 224-225)

Personal Care Products: Get EWG.ORG Skin Deep app and rate your cosmetics, hair supplies, lotions, makeup. Anything you apply to your skin hits your bloodstream within seconds. SUMMER EWG.ORG guide to a healthy summer. Read about bug repellents and sunscreens. If you are going to be in chlorine often, take a shower to saturate the skin prior to jumping in to reduce the chlorine absorption. After swimming, shower off well and consider using a gentle exfoliant to remove the chlorine.

Root Canals: Dr. Weston Price showed that many chronic degenerative diseases originate from root-filled teeth—the most frequent being the heart and circulatory diseases. He wrote two groundbreaking books in 1922 detailing his research into the link between dental pathology and chronic illness. Root canals and the jaw bone frequently harbor bacteria like MARCoNS (Multiple Antibiotic Coagulase Negative *Staphylococci*).

Amalgam Fillings: Find a biological dentist near you and learn how to safely remove the fillings that are leaching mercury into your body. A biological dentist is trained to remove the toxic substance and replace it with a biocompatible alternative.

Sleep & Relaxation Modifications

Sleep disturbance is multifactorial. Hormones, genetics, chronic stress, a restricted airway, sleep apnea, and pain can all be the root causes of insomnia and poor-quality sleep.

Our main objective to heal from chronic conditions is to remove as much burden from the body as possible. Sleep is often restored once we begin to practice preparing for sleep with good sleep hygiene, choose foods that are not igniting an inflammatory response, reduce our toxic exposure to harmful chemicals in common household items, balance hormones, and once we begin to hydrate and support our bodies with the medical and structural integrating pieces.

Most of the processes that occur in the mind and body follow natural rhythms. Those with a cycle length of about one day are called circadian rhythms. Your circadian system seems to be programmed to a large extent by genetics.

What Are Circadian Rhythms? Circadian rhythms have an effect on all of the following: body temperature, sleep, and wakefulness, and various hormonal changes. Your personalized care plan will be supporting your body to return it back to its natural circadian rhythm by addressing the emotional, environmental, lifestyle, nutrition, and genetic contributing factors.

Sleep Hygiene: Electronics are off at least an hour prior to bedtime. Practice affirmations and deep breathing, a dark room, and use an essential oil diffuser.

Transform Your Thoughts: your thoughts create feelings. What have you found to evaluate if your thoughts are serving you and how to reframe them so as to benefit you? We place so much pressure on ourselves. Did you know that a bald eagle catches one fish every eighteen attempts? Use the emotional scale and breathing exercises to reframe any perseverating thoughts which make falling asleep a challenge.

EMFs: electromagnetic fields. ElectromagneticHealth.org also offers free audio interviews with some of the world's leading experts in the field of EMF. You can learn about measuring instrumentation at www.emfsafetystore.com and www.bioinitiative.org. The TRIFIELD EMF meter model TF2 is an excellent tool.

Epsom Salt Baths: epsom salt is magnesium sulfate. Magnesium is a mineral that is very relaxing to the body. Many people have a deficiency in magnesium and sulfate. This can contribute to sleeping problems, behavioral issues, cramping muscles, and a tendency to just not feel well. This is important because sulfur chemistry is deeply connected to detoxification. The detoxification system in our body is critical to rid the body of toxins and we know that toxicity is a big problem.

Relationship Modifications

Conventional Medicine for chronic conditions has made us accept the belief that healing is outside of ourselves. Do you believe that it's the medical provider's responsibility to heal you? Do you believe that a pharmaceutical product (drug) will resolve your complaints and allow you to access good health and freedom? Functional medicine asks that healing is initiated from your mental, emotional, and spiritual health. Functional medicine asks you to assume a leadership role and accountability for the life you lead to reclaim your health and vitality. You are the hero of your story. The doctor is your guide. Your journey is about the relationship you have with facing your greatest challenges and rising to the occasion. Your relationship with yourself is a key indicator of health and well-being.

Self-Love: self-love is one of the most challenging lifestyle factors to master. This is largely because of belief systems that have either been given to us or that we have adopted along the way. Loving who you are at this exact moment, honoring the challenges and celebrating the triumphs that have brought you to this moment, evaluating your belief sets, and honoring who you are will influence your success. You cannot restore balance without self-love.

Beliefs: your thoughts create your words, which create your habits, which creates your character, which create your reality. Your beliefs are what drive your thoughts. And your thoughts drive your feelings. Evaluate your beliefs. Ask, "Is this true? Do I really believe this?" A compromised GI tract is going to alter your brain chemistry and self-sabotaging, self-defeating thoughts will be loud. Do you have to believe them?

> *"The greatest discovery of my generation is that human beings can alter their lives by altering their attitudes of mind."* William James

Gratitude: Robert A. Emmons, Ph.D, a leading scientific expert on gratitude, sees the practice of gratitude as having two components: affirming the goodness in our lives, and exploring where that goodness comes from. Check out viacharacter.org

Words Are Powerful: the words you choose such as *"I can't eat that,"* or *"I'm on a restricted diet,"* are phrases that will instigate others to feel defensive and, worse, hostile toward your functional medicine plan. How are you using the emotional scale and nonviolent communication to improve your communication?

Exercise & Movement Modifications

Examine your expectations and beliefs regarding exercise. Do you believe that "valuable" exercise must be intense?

It's easy to expect yourself to do more than what is reasonable.

If you are expecting more out of yourself than you are ready for, chances are you are avoiding exercise!

"What can I do today to add in more movement?" is a fantastic question to be asking yourself. If you are looking for it, you will find it.

As you go through your healing process you will feel like you have more energy to be more active. And as you budget your time and money to allow time to exercise, the better your healing results will be.

Start small and increase movement over time.

Gentle exercises like walking and yoga are just as beneficial as HIIT (high-intensity interval training) and other high-intensity workouts. A balanced approach is usually the best path forward.

Your provider can also give insight on what exercise is right for you, based on your genetic code.

Relaxation Choices: progressive muscle is one exercise to help induce relaxation. Beginning with the head, systematically relax each part of your body. Autogenics is a technique where you begin with the head, and imagine each part feeling warm and heavy. To practice a visual imagery relaxation technique, imagine a peaceful scene or location. A meditation practice can be repeating peaceful, single, syllable words like calm, peace, and joy. And a countdown relaxation technique is to count from one to ten as you inhale, and ten to one as you exhale.

Mindful Movement: yoga, qi gong, and tai chi are wonderful ways to learn a series of movements that are connected to breathing and mental practices. There are many health benefits ranging from improved lung function to better mental health.

Movement at Work: if you like app reminders, you will like StretchClock, DeskActive, BreakPal, and Office-Fit. Research exercises to do at work. Start a workout group. Corporate Wellness is on the rise. Microsoft is testing out the four-day workweek! Anything is possible.

Restorative Yoga: those healing from adrenal exhaustion is not going to benefit from vigorous movement. Restorative yoga, although not burning calories, has ample benefits worth investigating.

Working Out Strong Emotions: when you do X expecting Y and Y does not come quickly, you are more likely to stop doing X in a short period of time. Weight loss can take up to six months or, more realistically, longer to start seeing results. Make working out about more than losing weight. Make it about prevention from losing your mind! Make it about working out strong emotions that are toxic!

Exercise Guidelines: get at least 150 minutes of moderate aerobic activity or seventy-five minutes of vigorous aerobic activity three times a week, or a combination of moderate and vigorous activity. Add two days of strength training that make your muscles work harder than usual. Start with five minutes and work your way up!

(If you have a vector-borne illness, you should avoid aerobic exercise until you are almost finished with your treatment protocol.)

Body Image: Michelangelo is famous for saying that he worked to liberate the forms imprisoned in the marble. He saw his job as simply removing what was extraneous. Focus on the masterpiece that is your body rather than the extraneous flesh you are trying to lose.

Structural Integration Therapies

Exercise and bodywork are two of the best ways to support your detox pathways, support your digestion, and help shift your nervous system into the parasympathetic rest and digest setting.

With so much pressure and stress in today's world, we cannot heal if we remain locked in a flight-or-fight, otherwise known as, the sympathetic dominant nervous system.

Body care is not self-indulging, but rather a necessary component of your comprehensive care plan.

Visual Contrast Sensitivity Test (VCS Testing): VCS is often used as a nonspecific test of neurological function. Many things can affect the ability to perceive contrast. These include nutritional deficiencies, the consumption of alcohol, drug/medication use, and exposure to endogenous or exogenous neurotoxins and/or biotoxins, including volatile organic compounds (VOCs), venom from animal or insect stings or bites, some species of mold and the mycotoxins and microbial VOCs they produce, cyanobacteria, dinoflagellates (particularly Pfiesteria and Ciguatera), parasites, heavy metals like mercury and lead, and the pathogens responsible for Lyme disease and its common co-infections. For more information, see our research resources.

Go to www.vcstest.com and take the Online VCS screening test for each eye. Once you begin working with your medical provider you will UPLOAD the PDF result that was emailed to you AND send a secure message that the results have been uploaded into the patient portal. You need to pay the ten-dollar donation so that the full results will be emailed to you.

Baby Reflex Integration: Rhythmic Movement Training is a movement based, primitive (infant or neo-natal) reflex integration program that uses developmental movements, gentle isometric pressure and self-awareness to rebuild the foundations necessary to help overcome learning, sensory, emotional and behavioral challenges for children and adults. To learn more ask the Hope for Healing team about their handout.

Craniosacral Therapy (CST): craniosacral therapy is a form of bodywork that uses gentle touch to palpate the synarthrodial joints of the cranium. There are nerves that are not encased in bones and can be affected by inflammation and soft-tissue restriction. The cranial nerves are the nerves that regulate our senses and digestion.

Lymphatic Drainage Therapy: lymphatic drainage is relaxing and calming to the nervous system. In your body, your lymphatic system is the system responsible for eliminating cellular waste products and carrying them to the liver for detoxification. When your lymphatic system is not working properly, waste and toxins can build up and make you sick. Lymphatic congestion is a major factor leading to inflammation and disease.

Chiropractic Care: we are losing the cervical curve due to poor posture, cell phones, and too much desk work. This places strain on our nervous system. Chiropractors can feel aggressive. Be sure to communicate if the adjustments are too brutal.

Massage: often viewed as a luxury, this modality helps unlock the physical places we hold tension, therefore, unlocking the emotional vault that creates physical tension. We don't feel better by stuffing tension but rather by releasing it.

With so many modalities to choose from, and limited funds to afford organic foods, air, and water purifiers, supplements, labs, and functional medicine visits, it's okay to choose one intervention and have a session once a month for the next three months. Then you can choose another modality for the next three-month care plan you design.

Vision: is our dominant sense and primary source for gathering information in learning. 80 percent of what we learn is through our eyes, which means vision and/or visual perceptual difficulties can have a great effect on how we read, learn, and achieve in an academic setting.

A behavioral optometrist does more than assess 20/20 vision; the profession assesses how a person receives visual input from both eyes, and peripheral fields of vision, and how that input works together to improve how we process information.

An important characteristic of vision is binocular vision. Binocular vision is the ability to align both eyes on a visual point and combine the images seen by each eye into a single multidimensional image. Vision therapy can help patients with poor binocular coordination to train their eyes to work together in this way. This may significantly help improve your child's organization, focus, and attention to detail. When the binocular vision is unstable, it is very difficult to interpret the world. Information is coming in fragments, rather than a collection of information that paints a big picture. *Envisioning a Bright Future: Interventions That Work for Children and Adults with Autism Spectrum Disorders* by Patricia L. Lemer is recommended reading.

Here are some of the many conditions which can be positively affected by working with a behavioral optometrist for the right lenses and possibly vision therapy:

Amblyopia (lazy eye)
Amblyopia is the loss or lack of development of vision in (usually) one eye and is often associated with crossed eyes. The dysfunction actually occurs in the brain, not the eye itself, and is unrelated to any eye health problem. Amblyopia is not correctable with lenses but patients can benefit from vision therapy. Work to correct amblyopia can be started at any age but early detection and action offer the best chances for a complete cure.

Strabismus (eye turn)
Strabismus, a misalignment of the eyes, is a condition in which the eyes do not fixate as a pair. With strabismus, one eye can deviate inward, outward, or alternate, giving the person a "crossed" look and can frequently lead to amblyopia or "lazy eye." Although surgery is sometimes required to help "align" the eyes more closely, it only offers a cosmetic solution and does not result in functional improvement. The brain is what

controls eye alignment and if, for some reason, it does not fuse the images from the two eyes into one (creating a 3D picture), vision therapy can be used to train the brain to do so. As with many eye conditions, early detection and action will result in the best results.

Diplopia (double vision)

Diplopia is the result of both eyes independently focusing on different images as opposed to both images being fused into a single picture by the brain. There can be many possible causes for diplopia but, once the source is diagnosed, vision therapy can be very effective in correcting the condition.

Convergence Insufficiency

Convergence insufficiency occurs when your eyes do not properly align while focusing on a near object. When you read or look at a close object, your eyes should converge—turn inward together to align—resulting in a single image. Those who suffer from convergence insufficiency can experience double vision, strain, fatigue, and poor reading comprehension. This is a common problem in children who have reading difficulty in school and adults who find themselves transposing numbers. Vision therapy can greatly alleviate the symptoms that patients experience and can lead to more success in school, work, and everyday life.

Learning-Related Vision Difficulties

Difficulties in reading, writing, or learning can be the result of a vision problem. Many children diagnosed with learning disorders are experiencing them because of a vision-related problems, most of which can be greatly reduced through proper vision therapy.

Medical Section

"The doctor of the future will give no medicine but will interest his or her patients in the care of the human frame, in a proper diet, and in the cause and prevention of disease." Thomas Edison

This section is to prepare you for the conversations you may be having with your medical provider based on your or your child's lab results. This information is from Dr. Paula Kruppstadt MD, Chief Medical Officer at Hope for Healing. The practice cares for people from "womb to tomb." You can learn more at get2theroot.com

CIRS

Chronic inflammatory response syndrome (CIRS) is a condition that about a quarter of the population has worldwide. When a person with this condition is exposed to a biological toxin, they are unable to decrease the inflammation that the innate immune system generates. Your medical provider will identify if you have it and, if you do, the next step is to identify what can be done to balance your innate immune system. This is the part of the immune system that you're born with. Since there is no chronic inflammatory response ICD10 code, the code that is used is systemic inflammatory response syndrome without acute organ failure.

There are two types of immune systems, our innate immune system that we're born with and then our adaptive immune system. Our adaptive immune system produces antibodies when we are given vaccinations and when we are exposed to different things in the environment (such as viruses, bacteria, parasites, and fungi). The adaptive immune system mounts a response so we have antibodies to fight off infections, later on in life. If your innate immune system is on fire, then you should not have vaccinations while you're still in the throes of chronic inflammatory response syndrome.

Our medical providers recommend a blood panel ordered via LabCorp or Quest to evaluate your inflammatory markers.

We're going to do everything we can to help your environment be clean, because clean air, clean food, and clean water are very important to your ability to heal.

Microbial Dysbiosis GI Map Test

Dysbiosis is an imbalance in the natural flora of the digestive tract. Bacteria in the gut have the potential to overgrow which creates:

- Inflammation.
- Decreases nutrient absorption.
- And, in the case of autism, impair development.

By now, the majority of us have heard of parasites, yeast/fungi, *Clostridia*, viruses, and other bad bacteria (*H. pylori*) being hidden sources of inflammation. There is a method to clean up the gut. You have been introduced to the 5R approach, which is to remove, replace, reinoculate, repair, and and rebalance. That means, if there are any organisms in your gut that shouldn't be there, we want to get rid of them. Also, we don't kill our way to excellent health, but when you've got a pathogen living in your gut, you definitely have to eradicate it intelligently and safely.

At Hope for Healing, we use a stool test called the GI Map by Diagnostic Solutions. This is different from a stool culture because this is a DNA-based test. Other values are measured, such as blood, enzymes, and fecal secretory IgA. We glean great information from this test to guide your care and return the GI tract to a balanced, healthy state.

Mycotoxins

Mycotoxins are toxins produced by molds or fungi. Concentrations experienced in a home or building that has experienced water leaks are often high enough to trigger health responses in the occupants.

Dr. K talks about Biotoxin Illnesses

Biotoxin illnesses can be from bacteria, viruses, algae, venom from a snake-like copperheads, venom from spider bites, or mold in a home. 21 to 24 percent of the population has a genetic predisposition to developing biotoxin illness when they're exposed to a toxin of any kind.

Biotoxin illness is any illness that has the potential to cause a fever, like strep throat. Strep throat is caused by Group A Beta Hemolytic *Streptococci*. This bacteria has the potential to cause PANDAS.

We ask patients about the history of the home; like any water damage from floods, toilet overflowing, leaks from a dishwasher, sink, or a roof leak. It's important to share with your care team if the water damage lasted for more than forty-eight hours before the sheetrock was cut back. There are dry mold spores within regular sheetrock and if it's exposed to water, the spores will start to replicate and release mycotoxins.

If water damage is in your health history, there is a genetic test we will order to give insight if your genetics place you at risk to create inflammation in your body when exposed to a biotoxin. This involves HLA DR haplotype testing from LabCorp. The providers at Hope for Healing are qualified to interpret this test.

There are five different, separate genes HLA DRB1, DRB3, DRB4, DRB5, and DQB1. We calculate your risk using a website called myhousemakesmesick.com.

When we typically get sick, we get a fever, we feel bad, we're tired, then our temperature goes down and we feel better. The things in our body, immune molecules that make us feel bad, are called cytokines. Typically, cytokine levels will go down when an illness is over, but in someone who has a biotoxin illness, they won't go down back to normal and they will get sick. Typically, profound fatigue, brain fog, respiratory, mood, and gut problems will be present.

As far as mold goes, we get a lot of really good things from mold. We get antibiotics like penicillin, and we also have drugs that are called immunosuppressants. If cytokines, those little invisible messengers, stay elevated in our bodies, then our white cells don't know what to do. Our white cells help us fight off infections. The cytokines are like policemen. They tell the white cells what to do. If those white cells don't know what to do, then who knows what's going to happen when you're exposed to another biotoxin.

The majority of people tell me, "Well, I never get sick, but I don't feel well." Instead of feeling great, their level of functioning is low. They feel terrible, but they never get sick. In children with Autism, more often than not they don't get sick, but they are obviously not well—they are not meeting normal developmental milestones.

What are we going to do about this and why does this even matter? When we look at the biotoxin pathway, if you're one of those 21 to 24 percent of the population that is susceptible, then a cascade of events occurs in your body, leading to illness. We want to identify if you have this and help your immune system return to a balanced state.

Binders

A common term in functional medicine is **binders**. These are nutrients that go into your body and mop up toxic substrates. Examples of binders are cholestyramine, GI Detox+, and Standard Process okra pepsin E3.

Lyme Disease

We have observed in the clinical setting that mold toxins cause similar immune suppression as Lyme disease. Twenty-five percent of the population is sensitive to mold. It's common for Lyme patients' immune systems to handle the disease just fine until their bodies become overwhelmed by exposure to mold.

We feel it is nearly impossible to improve your Lyme symptoms if you don't resolve underlying immune suppression due to mold. In fact, mold toxin exposure can also suppress CD57 numbers just like Lyme does, so if exposed to mold, your numbers will be down even if you are doing a good job with treating Lyme disease. Lyme disease and coinfections are becoming more accepted as a root cause of today's common chronic and degenerative dis-eases. It's crucial to be sure you have done the nutrition, lifestyle, genetics, and medical intervention prerequisites before layering in a more advanced Lyme protocol. This is to strengthen your or your child's constitution to be strong enough to assist with this war to gain back control of the terrain.

Covid Tool Kit

If you are diagnosed with COVID-19, we have some recommendations to decrease inflammation in your body. To modulate many different inflammatory pathways in the body, many different supplements should be used. We have found the best success in our practice using aggressive use of PEA Soothe Support, Low Dose Naltrexone (prescription), pure cannabidiols in CBD products, Vitamin D3/K2, and Vitamin C at the onset of COVID-19. If you develop respiratory symptoms, you need a telemedicine or potentially an in-person appointment to have Azithromycin and Budesonide prescribed, if the medical provider believes these will be beneficial to you. To prevent the development of COVID-19 pneumonia, we are extremely aggressive whenever possible. For a COVID-19 Safety Kit at home, we recommend the following supplements. You may call our office to purchase and have these on hand, if you have not seen a medical provider yet.

The information is for informational purposes only, is not a substitute, and does not render medical or psychological advice, opinion, diagnosis, treatment, or cure. The information provided should not be used for diagnosing or treating a health problem or disease. It is not a substitute for professional care. Always seek the advice of your physician or other qualified healthcare providers with any questions you have regarding your medical conditions and treatment options.

Supplements

- PEA Soothe Support by Neurobiologix
- Waay CBD topical for kids or Medline oral CBD for adults
- Orthomune by Orthomolecular
- Oscillococcinum by Boiron
- Medline 2000 CBD with Myrcene
- Low Dose Naltrexone

Directions

- PEA Soothe Support by Neurobiologix (white):
  - **Children,** open up one half to one capsule, mix with food (it does not dissolve in liquid), and take twice a day (Please call Hope for Healing for the child's PEA product at 281-725-6767)
  - **Adults,** PEA Soothe Support (with resveratrol): take two to three capsules three times a day with water for up to three weeks, then go back down to one capsule twice a day (the higher dosing helps with brain inflammation!). PEA, Palmitoylethanolamide, decreases cytokine production in the brain and body.

- Orthomune by Orthomolecular (contains Vitamin C, Vitamin D, Zinc, Quercetin, and N-Acetyl-Cysteine)
  - **Children,** may take one capsule once a day until well.
  - **Adults,** take two capsules once a day.
- Oscillococcinum by Boiron: take one vial three times a day for two days at the onset of symptoms OR one vial a day after exposure to COVID-19.
  - This is the recommended dose for **both pediatrics and adults.**
- Waayb 5 mg/pump CBD (pure cannabidiols): **for children less than six years,** apply one pump to the base of the neck, just below the hairline, at bedtime, and rub in well.
- Waayb 10mg/pump CBD (pure cannabidiols): **for children greater than six** to twelve years, apply one pump to the base of the neck, just below the hairline, at bedtime, and rub in well.
- Medline 2000 CBD with Myrcene: **for twelve years to adult.** Take 0.5 to 1.0 milliliter at bedtime. Hold under tongue for approximately twenty seconds. The pure cannabidiols, along with the myrcene (a terpene), bind to CB1 and CB2 receptors and drive down cytokine production. This is helpful for sleep. Do not take in the morning.
- Low Dose Naltrexone: if you are already an established patient and have had an initial appointment with one of our medical providers, we can prescribe this for you. This is taken (capsule) or applied (cream) in the morning. It drives down cytokines produced by opioid receptors.

Bristol Stool Chart

Ken Heaton, MD, from the University of Bristol, developed the chart in 1997 with the help of sixty-six volunteers. They changed their diets, swallowed special marker pellets, and kept a diary about their bowel movements: weight, shape, and how often they went.

You will be using the scale to talk about shapes and types of poop, what doctors call stools. It's also known as the Meyers Scale. Typically, there are seven types. Ideally, you want to have type 3 or type 4. They are "perfect" stool shapes. Your poop should sink to the bottom of the toilet like a snake. It's a good idea to poop snakes, one to three times a day, that sink to the bottom of the toilet. If bowel movements are type 0-2 or types 5-7, then gut health is not optimal and the cause needs to be investigated.

Hope for Healing has modified the Bristol Stool Chart to include type zero. Dr. K added a type 0 to the scale: the Plum or Toilet Clogger. If your stool is type 1 or 2, you're probably constipated. types 5, 6, and 7 tend toward diarrhea.

Constipation

Constipation is caused by many things. It could be a lack of water intake, a lack of ingested fiber, a lack of physical movement, or a lack of mitochondrial and neurological support (Nerve Growth Factor/Brain Derived Neurotropic Factor from the brain) that precision genetics identify, to name a few.

Start with the basics:

Make sure your child is ingesting half of their body weight in pounds in ounces of water. (Example: your child weighs thirty pounds; therefore, they should be drinking fifteen ounces of water a day)

Increase their fiber: 1 cup of organic red raspberries has more fiber than any other fruit.

- Dr. K recommends that you take a look at the Anti-Anxiety Cookbook by Allie Miller, RD. There is a constipation puree in the back of the book that is great for children! Purchase a Squatty Potty and learn massage for constipation. Reference the Bibliography to find resources.

- **Adults:** Ascorbate C Cleanse. One of the best ways to clear constipation for **adults** is Vitamin C!
  - Use Vitamin C instead of Miralax to clean the stool burden out of your gut. We specifically use Perque Potent C Guard Powder ©≠, available from Hope for Healing (get2theroot.com):

Supplements Dr. K recommends and can be purchased by calling Hope for Healing at (281) 725-6767.

Diarrhea

Hope for Healing recommends the following. Both of these products contain immunoglobulins that bind toxins in the gut that lead to diarrhea.

- **Immune/GI Recovery Chewable (Neurobiologix)**©
  - Have your child chew one after each loose stool.

- **SBI Protect Powder (Orthomolecular)**©
  - Use one scoop in room temperature water after each loose stool.

Gut-Brain Axis Modulation

Over the past two decades, the gut-brain axis has become a heavily researched topic. The gut-microbiota-brain axis has been described as a multidirectional communication channel between the three systems: the gut, gut microbes, and the brain.

Although research is still substantiating the context in which the gut-brain axis contributes to treating psychiatric and gastrointestinal disorders, it is our experience that understanding the enteric nervous system (ENS), the vagus nerve, and digestion is important when pursuing root cause medicine.

First defined in 1921 by British physiologist John Langley, the **enteric nervous system (ENS)** is a network of sensory neurons, motor neurons, and interneurons embedded in the wall of the gastrointestinal system, extending from the lower third of the esophagus to the rectum. The term enteric nervous system was classified as a branch of the autonomic nervous system alongside the sympathetic and parasympathetic branches. Although capable of functioning independently of the CNS, the ENS works in concert with the other branches of the autonomic nervous system to coordinate digestive functions. The ENS is called the "second brain." The ENS is responsible for coordinating motor reflexes, controlling the exchange of water and electrolytes across the mucosal epithelium, regulating local blood flow, and regulating immunological processes.

The state of the enteric nervous system (ENS) determines the functioning of the digestive system. A parasympathetic state of ENS allows the proper functioning of the digestive tract. In particular, the vagus nerve plays an important role in activating digestion. Once the brain activates the vagus nerve, our body switches to the parasympathetic nervous response and starts digestion.

In the bibliography, you will find resources to learn more about this intrinsic neural control of gut functions involved in digestion and how the ENS interacts with the immune system, gut microbiota, and epithelium to maintain mucosal defense and barrier function.

Vagus Nerve

The vagus nerve is our X cranial nerve. It innervates most organs of our body, including our gut.

The vagus nerve represents the main component of the parasympathetic nervous system, which oversees a vast array of crucial bodily functions, including control of mood, immune response, digestion, and heart rate. The vagal nerves, a key part of your parasympathetic nervous system, carry signals between your brain, heart, and digestive system.

Vagal tone is correlated with one's capacity to regulate stress responses and can be influenced by breathing; its increase through meditation and yoga likely contributes to resilience and the mitigation of mood and anxiety symptoms.

Vagus nerve damage can lead to gastroparesis, which means food not moving into your intestines. When someone gags easily, has difficulty swallowing capsules, and has constipation, Dr. K has learned this is an indicator that the vagus nerve is under stimulated. The body is in fight or flight mode (sympathetic overdrive).

Dr. K's recommendations:
You can gargle with water and change the sound of your voice/gargling "aggressively," sing loud and if you can, gag yourself (but hopefully without throwing up).

Children can practice blowing bubbles, blowing a pinwheel, and also singing loudly/dance, and can also gargle loudly with water. Parents need to demonstrate this—make it fun, and all the while, your children are stimulating their vagus nerve, and it also helps move stool through the bowel more easily!

Dr. K also recommends using tongue twisters by looking at Rodney Saulsberry's *Tongue Twister and Vocal Warm-Ups*. Also, look at *99 Tortuous Tricky Tough Tongue Twisters*. Since the vagus nerve is a cranial nerve, which means it is not encased in bone, Cranio Sacral Therapy is also an intervention to consider when deciding to stimulate the function of the vagus nerve.

Dr. K says if you do these vagus nerve exercises several times a day, this can help improve your digestion and brain health and provide some balancing of your autonomic nervous system.

Dr. K also recommends the book *Accessing the Healing Power of the Vagus Nerve: Self-Help Exercises for Anxiety, Depression, Trauma, and Autism* by Stanley Rosenberg.

Puberty

It's absolutely imperative to move your child into inflammation control in the prepubescent and pubertal years!

If your preteen or teen is aggressive or very emotional, use PEA 2-3 caps 3 times daily until the symptoms subside. Optimizing their anti-inflammatory control utilizing pure cannabidiols (CBD products), omega-3 fatty acids, low-dose naltrexone, sleep (are they sleeping well?), and throwing out the electronic screen devices (video games) will all help them traverse the volatile and tumultuous pubescent years with more grace. Ensure they have many physical activity outlets and that you work closely with your functional medicine provider to layer in adequate methylation support appropriately. Methylation need skyrockets at about age 8 years and continues to increase until about 19 to 24 years of age and levels out until you reach ~64 years of age. At this age, it is important to work with a functional medicine provider to support methylation again.

Eczema

What is eczema? With atopic dermatitis, the biggest culprit is diet. Another big culprit is a lack of the proper types of omega-three fatty acids (fish oil) and a lack of glutathione in the skin.

Glutathione

Glutathione, (pronounced gloota-thigh-own) is a buzzword. It is the body's most important molecule to prevent disease and stay healthy. It's the master anti-inflammatory and master antioxidant. It's *made* in our body, but some people have "faulty" glutathione production or just don't make enough. Glutathione is composed of three amino acids: **cysteine, glutamic acid, and glycine.** Without enough glutathione, we can never recover from chronic disease. If you don't make enough because of genetic issues, then you need to take oral glutathione and/or have it IV. You can also help your body have the building blocks to make it by consuming foods high in the amino acids that make glutathione. Some great sulfur-rich food choices to boost your glutathione production are as follows: onions, garlic, and cruciferous vegetables like cabbage, cauliflower, broccoli, kale, and collard greens.

High Blood Pressure

In functional medicine, we look for why the person has high blood pressure rather than simply at what can be done to lower it; it's a person-centered approach, versus a disease-centered one. Factors to consider include genetic predispositions, nutritional deficiencies, environmental triggers, and lifestyle habits, such as

- Deficiencies in nutrients such as biotin, vitamin D, vitamin C, B1, choline, **magnesium,** and CoQ10.
- Toxic levels of mercury.
- Hypothyroidism: appropriate management of a thyroid condition such as autoimmune thyroiditis can normalize blood pressure.
- A lack of dietary potassium and too much sodium. Balancing these nutrients can help balance blood pressure.

- Magnesium deficiency. Many people are deficient in magnesium, which can help relax the blood vessels. (Adults should try Triple Mag Plus, 3 capsules twice a day, available in our supplement store, to lower their blood pressure.)
- Chronic systemic inflammation.
- Elevated blood sugar and metabolic syndrome (pre-diabetes), are related to hypertension.
- Hormonal imbalances, such as estrogen deficiency, can lead to high blood pressure.

By addressing these and other factors, a functional medicine approach addresses the root cause of high blood pressure. Research has shown that up to 62 percent of high blood pressure patients were able to go off their antihypertensive medications and maintain normal blood pressure by making diet and lifestyle changes.

Eating a whole-foods, vegetable-based diet and avoiding processed foods and layering the interventions suggested in our comprehensive care plan will help keep you sufficient and balanced in the right minerals to support healthy blood pressure.

Ask about the Cardiometabolic Food Plan designed by Functional Medicine Practitioners.

What is Detoxification?

A person's toxic body burden is a result of three main factors.

First, there is the toxicant exposure we each may have received from both internal and external sources, as previously discussed.

Second, each person's genetic predisposition to effectively produce detoxification enzymes for processing these compounds or substrates is unique and depends on familial influence.

Last, the integration of proper nutrition and ongoing dietary ingestion of helpful detoxification nutrients or phytonutrients can impact the body's capacity to appropriately reduce the presence of toxicants and lower the body's burden.

Recommended Resources

Reading Recommendations

QUICK TIP: If you don't enjoy reading, downloading an app like Audible to listen to the books below is a great alternative.

- *Mold Illness: Surviving and Thriving: A Recovery Manual for Patients & Families Impacted by CIRS* by Paula Vetter, RN, MSN, FNP-C, Laurie Rossi, RN, Cindy Edwards, CBA
  - Mold & biotoxin illness

- *Mold Warriors: Fighting America's Hidden Health Threat* by Ritchie C. Shoemaker, James Schaller, Patti Schmidt
  - Mold & biotoxin illness

- *Gratitude Journal* by Kurzgesagt
  - Mental & emotional health

- *The Disease Delusion: Conquering the Causes of Chronic Illness for a Healthier, Longer, and Happier Life* by Jeffrey Bland, MD
  - Functional medicine

- *Tiny Habits: The Small Changes That Change Everything* by BJ Fogg, Ph.D
  - Lifestyle improvement

- *Soul of Shame: Retelling the Stories we Believe About Ourselves* by Curt Thompson, MD
  - Trauma recovery

- *Too Perfect: When Being in Control Gets out of Control* by Allan Mallinger, MD, Jeannette DeWyze
  - Mental & emotional health

- *The Ruthless Elimination of Hurry: How to stay emotionally healthy and spiritually alive in the chaos of the modern world* by John Mark Comer
  - Spirituality

- *Searching for Enough: The High-Wire Walk Between Faith and Doubt* by Tyler Staton
  - Spirituality

- *Food: What the Heck Should I Eat?* by Mark Hyman, MD
  - Nutrition

- *The Wahls Protocol: A Radical New Way To Treat All Chronic Autoimmune Conditions Using Paleo Principles* by Terry Wahls, MD
  - Nutrition

- *The 5 Love Languages: The Secret to Love That Lasts* by Gary Chapman
  - Relationships & community

- *Why Emotions Matter: Recognize Your Body Signals. Grow in Emotional Intelligence. Discover an Embodied Spirituality* by Tristen K Collins, LPC and Jonathan Collins, with Melissa Binder
  - Emotional health

- *The Ozone Miracle: How You Can Harness the Power of Oxygen to Keep You and Your Family Healthy* by Frank Shallenberger, MD
  - Ozone

- *The Body Keeps Score: Brain, Mind, and Body in the Healing of Trauma* by Bessel Van Der Kolk, MD
  - Trauma recovery

- *Solve Your Child's Sleep Problems* by Richard Ferber, MD
  - Sleep

- *Limitless: Upgrade Your Brain, Learn Anything Faster, and Unlock Your Exceptional Life* by Jim Kwik
  - Mental & emotional health

- *The Healing Code: 6 Minutes to Heal the Source of Your Health, Success, or Relationship* by Alexander Loyd, PhD
  - Whole body health

- *DIY Natural Household Cleaners* by Matt and Betsy Jabs at diynatural.com
  - Homemade cleaning products

- *The Autoimmune Fix: How to Stop the Hidden Autoimmune Damage That Keeps You Sick, Fat, and Tired Before It Turns Into Disease* by Dr. Tom O'Bryan, DC
  - Homemade cleaning products
  - Whole body health
  - Autoimmunity

- *The Good Gut: Taking Control of Your Weight, Your Mood, and Your Long-term Health* by Justin Sonnenburg, Erica Sonnenburg
  - Gut health

- *Brain Maker: The Power of Gut Microbes to Heal and Protect Your Brain for Life* by David Perlmutter and Kristin Loberg
  - Gut health

- *The Microbiome Solution: A Radical New Way to Heal Your Body from the Inside Out* by Dr. Robynne Chutkan MD
  - Gut health

- *The Gut Balance Revolution: Boost Your Metabolism, Restore Your Inner Ecology, and Lose the Weight for Good!* by Gerard E. Mullin
  - Gut health

- *The Second Brain: A Groundbreaking New Understanding of Nervous Disorders of the Stomach and Intestine* by Michael Gershon
  - Gut health

- *Accessing the Healing Power of the Vagus Nerve: Self-Help Exercises for Anxiety, Depression, Trauma, and Autism* by Stanley Rosenberg.
  - Vagus Nerve

- *Anti-Anxiety Cookbook* by Allie Miller, RD
  - Mood, Elimination

- *Infinite Potential: What Quantum Physics Reveals About How We Should Live* by Lothar Schafer
  - Quantum Physics

- *The Emotion Code: How to Release Your Trapped Emotions for Abundant Health, Love, and Happiness* by Dr. Bradley Nelson and Tony Robbins
  - Emotional Intelligence

- *Envisioning a Bright Future: Interventions That Work for Children and Adults with Autism Spectrum Disorders* by Patricia L. Lemer
  - Vision

- *Breaking the Habit of Being Yourself* by Joe Dispenza, Adam Boyce, et al.
  - Metacognition, Neuroplasticity

- *Character Strengths and Virtues: A Handbook and Classification 1st Edition* by Christopher Peterson
  - Positive Psychology

- *Positive Intelligence: Why Only 20% of Teams and Individuals Achieve Their True Potential AND HOW YOU CAN ACHIEVE YOURS* by Shirzad Chamine
  - Emotional Intelligence

- *No Grain, No Pain: A 30-Day Diet for Eliminating the Root Cause of Chronic Pain* by Peter Osborne

- *Motivational Interviewing with Adolescents and Young Adults* by Sylvie Naar and Mariann Suarez.

Website and Video Content

- The third-leading cause of death in the US most doctors don't want you to know about.
  - https://www.cnbc.com/2018/02/22/medical-errors-third-leading-cause-of-death-in-america.html

- Broaden-and-Build Theory of Positive Emotions by Dr. Barbara Fredrickson
  - https://positivepsychology.com/broaden-build-theory/

- Why Gratitude is Good
  - https://greatergood.berkeley.edu/article/item/why_gratitude_is_good

- The Gene-ius Within: Unlocking the Beneficial Effects of Heart-Focused Intention on Gene Expression
  - https://www.heartmath.org/resources/videos/gene-ius-within/

- Surviving Mold: Actino Central
  - https://www.survivingmold.com/legal-resources/actino-central

- Evidence is the Loudest Voice
  - https://drjoedispenza.com/pages/scientific-research

- The bowel and beyond: the enteric nervous system in neurological disorders
  - https://www.nature.com/articles/nrgastro.2016.107

- The enteric nervous system
  - https://pubmed.ncbi.nlm.nih.gov/36521049/

- Vagus Nerve as Modulator of the Brain–Gut Axis in Psychiatric and Inflammatory Disorders
  - https://www.ncbi.nlm.nih.gov/pmc/articles/PMC5859128/

- Probiotics and gut-brain axis modulation
  - https://www.sciencedirect.com/topics/agricultural-and-biological-sciences/enteric-nervous-system

- The Gut-Microbiota-Brain Axis in Autism Spectrum Disorder
  - https://www.ncbi.nlm.nih.gov/books/NBK573606/

- Squatty Potty
  - https://bit.ly/3Lj3xW2
  - Picture of child using Squatty Potty: https://www.pinterest.com/pin/447404544204876419

- Massage for constipation.
  - Here is a link to a massage for constipation that I find very helpful: https://www.youtube.com/watch?v=5XGwvPoiItw

- Bio resonance sound healing: https://vocalanalysis.net/

- Energy work: https://arielenergyhealer.com/

Podcast Recommendations

- Dr. Mark Hyman: The Doctor's Farmacy
  - All things functional medicine

- Caroline Leaf: Cleaning Up the Mental Mess
  - Practical and scientific tips to take back control over mental, emotional, and physical health

- Bridgetown Audio Podcast
  - Spirituality and health

- What the Func?!
  - Functional medicine

- Coffee with Dr. Stewart
  - Genetics and functional medicine

- Dhru Purohit Podcast
  - All things functional medicine
  - Alternative Health

- BetterHealthy Guy Blogcasts: Empowering Your Better Health
  - Alternative Health

Books

Prochaska, Dr. James, and Prochaska, Dr. Janice. *Changing to Thrive: Using the Stages of Change to Overcome the Top Threats to Your Health and Happiness* Hazelden September 2016

Comer, John Mark. *The Ruthless Elimination of Hurry: How to stay emotionally healthy and spiritually alive in the chaos of the modern world* WaterBrook (October 29, 2019)

Hicks, Esther, and Jerry. *The Astonishing Power of Emotions: Let Your Feelings Be Your Guide* Hay House, Incorporated September 2007

Noricks, Jay. *Parts Psychology: A Trauma-Based, Self-State Therapy for Emotional Healing* New University Press, September 9, 2011,

Tarragona, Margarita, Ph.D. *Positive Identities: Narrative Practices and Positive Psychology (The Positive Psychology Workbook Series),* CreateSpace Independent Publishing Platform, March 22, 2013,

Bibliography

Website Content and Videos

- Urbina, Ian. "Think Those Chemicals Have Been Tested?" April 13, 2013,
  - https://www.nytimes.com/2013/04/14/sunday-review/think-those-chemicals-have-been-tested.html

- Environmental Working Group, EWG "Body Burden: The Pollution in Newborns" July 14, 2005,
  - https://www.ewg.org/research/body-burden-pollution-newborns
  - ewg.org/guides/cleaners
  - EWG Healthy Living app
  - EWG's Healthy Living Home Guide
    - https://www.ewg.org/healthyhomeguide/

- Think Dirty App.com

- John Bower Founder, Healthy House Institute Healthy House Reference Manual. "Chapter 5: Indoor Air Pollutants and Toxic Materials"
  - https://www.cdc.gov/nceh/publications/books/housing/cha05.htm

- Medicine LibreTexts 1.1B: Defining Physiology
  - (1.1B: Defining Physiology - Medicine LibreTexts)

- Joshua Schultz, Psy.D "Your Complete Nonviolent Communication Guide"
  - https://positivepsychology.com/non-violent-communication/

- Visual Contrast Sensitivity Test Online Contrast Sensitivity Test, OCST, and OCSTPro are trademarks of VCSTest.com.
  - https://vcstesting.com

- Copyright 2008, Royal College of Nursing. "Irritable Bowel Syndrome in Adults: Diagnosis and Management of Irritable Bowel Syndrome in Primary Care"
  - https://www.ncbi.nlm.nih.gov/books/NBK51939/

- The VIA Character. "Strengths Survey Get to Know Your Greatest Strengths."
  - https://viacharacter.org

- Mann, Leon. "Studies in Curriculum Decision Making: A Conflict Theory Approach. Final Report."
  - https://files.eric.ed.gov/fulltext/ED070030.pdf

- Warner, Judith. "Concocting a Cure for Kids With Issues" March 10, 2010,
  - https://www.nytimes.com/2010/03/14/magazine/14vision-t.html
- Dos Santos Rodrigues, Livia. "Jarisch-Herxheimer reaction in a patient with syphilis and human immunodeficiency virus infection" December 2018
  - https://www.researchgate.net/publication/329410187
- Dr. Peter Gibson and Dr. Sue Shepherd "Low FODMAP Diet"
  - https://shepherdworks.com.au/disease-information/low-fodmap-diet/
- Institute of Functional Medicine
  - IFM.org
- Dave Ramsey Financial Peace
  - https://www.ramseysolutions.com/ramseyplus/financial-peace/home
- Every Dollar budget app
  - https://www.ramseysolutions.com/ramseyplus/everydollar
- Well Screened EMF products
  - www.emfsafetystore.com
- A Rationale for Biologically-Based Exposure Standards for Low-Intensity Electromagnetic Radiation
  - www.bioinitiative.org
- Electronic Magnetic Health
  - ElectromagneticHealth.org
- Weil, Dr. Andrew. Three Breathing Exercises And Techniques
  - https://www.drweil.com/health-wellness/body-mind-spirit/stress-anxiety/breathing-three-exercises/
- Egnew, Thomas. *The Meaning of Healing: Transcending Healing,* The National Library of Medicine.
  - https://www.ncbi.nlm.nih.gov/pmc/articles/PMC1466870/
- Klein, Kendall, Tougas. Changing Brains, Changing Lives: Researching the Lived Experience of Individuals Practicing Self-Directed Neuroplasticity
  - https://sophia.stkate.edu/cgi/viewcontent.cgi?article=1019&context=ma_hhs
- Hanson, Rick. The Practical Science of Lasting Happiness
  - https://www.rickhanson.net/
- The Transtheoretical Model (TTM)
  - https://www.prochange.com/transtheoretical-model-of-behavior-change

- Internal Family Systems by Dick Schwartz
  - https://ifs-institute.com/

- The Stretch Clock.com
  - StretchClock reminds you to stretch and guides you through easy exercises you can do at the desk

- Tate, Robert. The Magic Pill Documentary
  - https://www.imdb.com/title/tt6035294/

About the Author

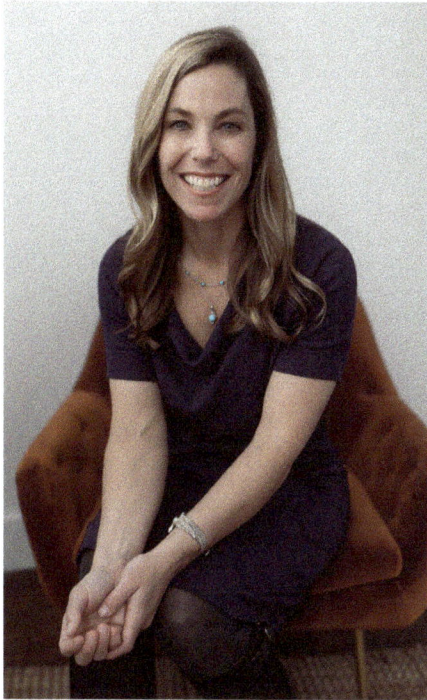

Kara Ware, a National Board and Functional Medicine Health Coach, has spent nearly two decades healing her son of the underlying causes creating the symptoms commonly referred to as Autism.

She did not accept the limiting belief there was nothing she could do for her son. Her son looked like he was in unbearable pain. She knew there must be something she could do to help him feel better, and therefore, behave better.

In times of dial-up internet and flip phones that did not text, let alone take photos and videos, she was divinely guided to learn about the sources of inflammation that were causing his pain and intolerable and terrifying Autistic behaviors and symptoms and how to intelligently and safely layer interventions to work in combination.

Kara discovered there were even more underlying conditions than Leaky Gut, Vitamin and Mineral Depletion, Microbial Overload, Suppressed Immune System, Heavy Metal and Mold Toxicity, Lyme Disease, etc.

She found her thoughts, which created her words, and then her actions which created her habits, which then created an atmosphere of healing was what ultimately allowed Kara to accomplish what many say is impossible.

When her perspective changed, and her anger turned to embracing what this journey had come to teach, the healing began. She learned her son came to teach her this shift from fear to love and how to support her family to thrive in today's environment.

This workbook is the accumulation of what Kara found and was willing to do to heal her son from this once thought dead-end diagnosis. Many pieces may seem insignificant; however, when all the nutrition and lifestyle and genetics and medical changes are layered in overtime to work in combination, and when love is the motivator, and the home becomes the headquarters for healing, miracles will happen.

www.ingramcontent.com/pod-product-compliance
Lightning Source LLC
Chambersburg PA
CBHW041427270326
41932CB00030B/3485